Adequacy of Sample Size in Health Studies

Adequacy of Sample Size in Health Studies

Stanley Lemeshow
David W. Hosmer Jr
Janelle Klar
University of Massachusetts

and

Stephen K. Lwanga
World Health Organization

Published on behalf of the World Health Organization by

JOHN WILEY & SONS
Chichester · New York · Brisbane · Toronto · Singapore

Published by John Wiley & Sons Ltd.
        Baffins Lane, Chichester
        West Sussex PO19 1UD, England

Distributed in the United States of America, Canada and
Japan by Alan R. Liss Inc., 41 East 11th Street, New York,
NY 10003, USA.

Library of Congress Cataloging-in-Publication Data

Adequacy of sample size in health studies / by Stanley Lemeshow...
  [et al.]
      p.   cm.
    Includes bibliographical references.
    ISBN 0 471 92517 9
      1. Public health—Research—Statistical methods.   2. Sampling
  (Statistics)   I. Lemeshow, Stanley.   II. World Health Organization.
    [DNLM: 1. Research Design. 2. Sampling Studies. WA 20.5 A232]
  RA440.85.A34   1990
  362.1′072—dc20
  DNLM/DLC
  for Library of Congress   89-22495
                                                                        CIP

British Library Cataloguing in Publication Data

Adequacy of sample size in health studies.
  1. Public health. Research techniques
  I. Lemeshow, Stanley   II. World Health Organisation
  363′.072

  ISBN 0 471 92517 9

Printed and bound by Courier International Ltd, Tiptree, Colchester

Table of Contents

Part II   Foundations of Sampling and Statistical Theory

Part III Tables for Sample Size Determination

Preface

The World Health Organization (WHO) Expert Committee on Health Statistics, in its tenth report (Technical Report Series, number 336 of 1966), concluded that in view of the important role played by sampling in many types of public health investigations and the shortage of experts in the theory and practice of sampling, epidemiologists and other health workers should be provided with facilities for obtaining a basic knowledge of sampling principles and methods and acquainted with their potential applications in the medical field. The Committee therefore recommended that a manual dealing with the general principles of sampling and describing in some detail the special problems and opportunities in the medical field would be a useful guide for many workers in public health. The manual would assist the statistician or sampling expert with no previous experience of medical applications, and would also prove valuable for training courses.

In 1973 a document: Adequacy of sample size (HSM/73.1) was issued by WHO's Statistical Methodology Unit, as a second edition of a 1961 document (MHO/PA/220.63) with reconstructed tables. Since then the document has been in steady demand. The 1973 document was issued by the then Health Statistical Methodology Unit of WHO in Geneva because "WHO (was) sponsoring a major program in medical research and workers engaged in it needed to have at their elbow a document answering questions on the adequacy of sample size". The current emphasis of the Organization's activities is different to that in 1973. While the tables in HSM/73.1 are still adequate for most purposes of experimental research, they do not cover important areas of case-control type studies and cluster sampling. These approaches are the most likely to be adopted by health managers in evaluating and monitoring their health programs.

WHO's Unit of Epidemiological and Statistical Methodology (ESM), in collaboration with the Organization's programs of: Diarrhoeal Disease Control (CDD), Expanded Immunization (EPI) and Research and Training in Tropical Diseases (TDR), sponsored the preparation of this book on the determination of adequate sample sizes under different situations. A number of "typical" questions which health workers pose to the statisticians concerning the size of the sample of subjects they should study are covered in this book. It is hoped that the book will meet the needs of health workers and managers faced with the problem of deciding how large a sample to survey or study, and that it will provide insight into the methodology of solving the most common problems of sample size needs.

The authors would like to acknowledge the editorial assistance of James L. Duppenthaler, World Health Organization, in the preparation of this work.

Introduction

The role of sampling in the health field

For most studies, especially those of human populations, all the people cannot be studied. This may be because the population is too large and therefore impossible to study every person due to time, financial and other resource constraints, or because it cannot be defined uniquely in either time or space. In such situations only a part of the population, a sample, would be studied and the results generalized to cover the whole population. It is the need to generalize the results based on the sample to the population that dictates the use of appropriate sampling techniques. Different samples drawn from the same population would give different results if the population elements are not identical. The variability of the sample results depends directly on the variability of the population elements and inversely on the size of the sample. Since human populations are so variable, sampling errors must be accepted as part of the study outcome.

A conscientious health worker planning a survey or a study will ask an apparently straightforward question: *How large a sample do I need?* Very often an immediate answer will be expected without realizing that a realistic answer has to be computed based on the specific aims of the survey or study. Additional information is therefore always required. A reasonable guess the expected result is usually a prerequisite for arriving at a satisfactory estimate of sample size. The health worker also has to indicate the required precision and the confidence with which the results are to be established, the operational constraints and any available information on the expected outcome.

The adequacy of any sample size is judged according to the scope of the survey or study results. For example, the question of sample size might not arise if one wants to study the efficacy of a rabies treatment drug, but it would be important to have an 'adequate' sample when one is testing a new anti-malaria drug. In the first example a positive result based even on a single case would be important since there is as yet no known cure for the disease. In the second example since there are known efficacious preventive measures the results of the new drug have to be based on a sufficiently large number of responses.

The size of the survey or study will naturally depend on the subject matter and the aims of the exercise, the desired precision etc. The collected information on the outcome can, however, be classified into different categories. Firstly, the outcome may be split into two categories; for example, disabled/not disabled, vaccinated/not vaccinated, existence of a health committee/lack of a health committee, etc. Secondly, the outcome may have a number of mutually exclusive and exhaustive possibilities; for example, attitudes, religious beliefs, blood groups, etc. In these two cases the data are generally summarized by percentages or rates. Thirdly, for each respondent (study subject) some numerical measurement may be recorded; for example, weight, age, height, blood pressure, body temperature etc. In this case the data are summarized by means (averages) and variances or their derivatives. Determination of sample size has to take into account the category into which the outcome falls.

When deciding on the size of the sample to use it should be realized that *absolute* sample size is more important than sample size *relative* to the whole population, in reducing sample variances when one is not dealing with very small populations. It is therefore very often better not to aim at, for example, increasing the sample from 5% of the population to say 10% but rather think in terms of absolute increments.

When data are to be analyzed in subgroups, for example by regions, the sampling errors of the subgroups are likely to be larger than the estimated errors for the whole sample since, by definition, subgroups are smaller. The larger the number of subdivisions, the smaller the sample sizes would be for the individual subgroups and hence the larger the sampling variations are likely to become, leading to less reliable population subgroup estimates.

The scope of this book

This book is divided into two parts. The first part gives solutions to typical problems and tables of minimum sample sizes for various survey and study designs, with the corresponding formulae. The second part gives a concise exposition of the theory behind the process of determining sample sizes. The first part may be looked at as the *application* section, and the second part as the *theoretical* section. The application section can be used without reference to the theoretical part. The cross references given are intended to assist the user of the book who is interested in knowing *why* the sample sizes are what they are said to be.

In the application section, tables are given for the estimation of proportions for longitudinal and cross-sectional studies and also for the comparison of two proportions. Corresponding tables are given for case-control studies. Included in this section are also tables for lot quality assurance surveys.

The second part of the book givesthe theoretical background to sample size determination covering populations, samples and their sampling distributions. It also covers characteristics of estimates of population parameters, hypothesis testing and two-sample confidence intervals, epidemiological study designs, basic sampling concepts and lot quality assurance sampling strategies. Sample size needs for measurements are given with the relevant formulae.

Methods of sample size determination which do not use the normal approximation to the exact distribution can be extremely complex, and are thus beyond the mathematical level of the proposed users of this book. Uses of the normal approximation in those instances in this book, when an exact analysis would theoretically be appropriate, are few in number and the resultant error in sample size arising from use of the normal approximation will be small. For these reasons no material which uses exact distributions is included.

Illustrative examples have been kept as simple as possible so as to be readily understandable by all users of the book.

This is a book on sample size determination, not a book on epidemiology. Many interesting epidemiological aspects of the illustrative examples are, therefore, not discussed.

Part I
Statistical Methods for Sample Size Determination

1 The one-sample problem

Estimating the population proportion

The true but unknown proportion in the population is denoted by P. The sampling distribution[a] of the sample proportion "p" is approximately normal with mean:[b] $E(p)=P$, and variance:[c] $Var(p)=P(1-P)/n$. The sampling distribution may be represented as in Fig. 1.

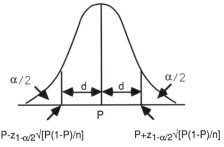

$\alpha/2$ d   d $\alpha/2$

P

$P-z_{1-\alpha/2}\sqrt{[P(1-P)/n]}$ $P+z_{1-\alpha/2}\sqrt{[P(1-P)/n]}$

Fig. 1 Sampling distribution of the sample proportion

The quantity d denotes the distance, in either direction, from the population proportion and may be expressed as

$$d = z_{1-\alpha/2}\sqrt{[P(1-P)/n]}$$

The quantity z represents the number of standard errors away from the mean. The quantity d is termed the *precision*[d] and can be made as small as desired by simply increasing the sample size n. Specifically, if z is chosen to be 1.960, then 95% of all sample proportions will fall within 1.960 standard errors of the population proportion P, where a standard error equals $\sqrt{P(1-P)/n}$. Unfortunately, this standard error is a function of the unknown population parameter P. Solving the above expression for n gives:

$$n = \frac{z_{1-\alpha/2}^2 P(1-P)}{d^2} \tag{1}$$

However, it should be notethat P(1-P) takes on the following values for different choices of P:

[a] See pages 55-60
[b] See page 57
[c] See pages 50-54
[d] See page 63

P	P(1-P)
0.5	0.25
0.4	0.24
0.3	0.21
0.2	0.16
0.1	0.09

The sample size selected will be largest when P equals 0.5, which is not an unreasonable level to use since P(1-P) decreases rather slowly as the difference between P and 0.5 increases.

Hence, it is recommended that when the researcher has no idea as to what the level of P is in the population, choosing 0.5 for P in the formula for sample size will always provide enough observations, irrespective of the actual value of the true proportion. In such circumstances, the following formula should be used in order to estimate the population proportion to within d percentage points of the true P:

$$n = z^2_{1-\alpha/2} \, [0.25]/d^2 \qquad\qquad (1a)$$

Tables 1a-1c present sample sizes for z = 1.645 (90% confidence), 1.960 (95% confidence), and 2.576 (99% confidence) for d ranging from 0.01 to 0.25, and for P ranging from 0.05 to 0.90 in increments of 0.05. These alternative levels are presented for P since there are some situations where the researcher has a reasonable idea as to the actual value. For example, if the rate to be estimated is the infant death rate, using P=0.5 would clearly yield much too large a sample size.

Example I.1.1
A district medical officer seeks to estimate the proportion of children in the district receiving appropriate childhood vaccinations. Assuming a simple random sample of a community is to be selected, how many children must be studied if the resulting estimate is to fall within *10 percentage points* of the true proportion with 95% confidence?

Solution
Using formula (1a), n = (1.960)^2(0.25)/(0.10)^2 = 96.04 and rounding up to the nearest integer, a sample of 97 children would be needed in order to be 95% confident of estimating the population proportion of children appropriately vaccinated. This value may also be found in Table 1b under the column headed 0.50 and in the row headed 0.10. As can be seen in that table, any value for the population proportion other than 0.5 would have required a *smaller* sample size. Hence, use of 0.5 as the value of P in the formula provides a *conservative* estimate of the required sample size. As can be seen from Tables 1a-1c, as the desired confidence increases, the required sample size also increases (a minimum sample size 167 would be required for 99% confidence).

Example I.1.2
A local health department wishes to estimate the prevalence rate of tuberculosis among children under five years of age in its locality. How many children should be included in the sample so that the rate may be estimated to within 5 percentage points of the true value with 99% confidence?

Solution

From Table 1a with P=0.5 and d=0.05, it can be seen that a sample of 666 children should be studied. If, however, the health department knows that the rate does not exceed 20%, a sample of size 427 would be necessary. If studying this many children is unrealistic with respect to time and money, the investigators should lower their requirements of confidence to, perhaps, 90% . In this case Table 1c shows that for d=0.05 and P=0.20, a sample size of only 174 is necessary.

Example I.1.3

A new treatment has cured three out of ten cases of a previously fatal disease. How many cases must be treated in order to be 95% confident that the recovery rate with the new treatment lies between 25% and 35%?

Solution

In Table 1b, using the column headed 0.30 and the row headed 0.05 it can be seen that the necessary sample size is 323 cases.

·

In Example I.1.1, it should be noted that 97 is the requirement if *simple random sampling*[e] is to be used. This would never be the case in an actual field survey. As a result, the sample size would go up by the amount of the "design effect"[f]. For example, if cluster sampling[g] were to be used, the design effect might be estimated as 2. This means that in order to obtain the same precision, twice as many individuals must be studied with cluster sampling as with the simple random sampling strategy. Hence, 184 subjects would be required.

It might seem more reasonable, in the same example, to require the estimate of $\overset{\bullet}{P}$ to fall within 10% of P rather than to within 10 percentage points of P. For example, if the true proportion vaccinated was 0.20, the strategy used in the above example would result in estimates falling between 0.10 and 0.30 in 95 out of every 100 samples drawn from this population. Instead, if we require our estimate to fall within 10% of 0.20, we would find that 95 out of every 100 samples would result in estimates between 0.20+0.1(0.20) = 0.22 and 0.20-0.1(0.20) = 0.18. To derive the expression appropriate for this formulation of the problem, we adopt the approach used by Levy and Lemeshow[42].

Let θ be the unknown population parameter as before and let $\hat{\theta}$ be the estimate of θ. Let ε, the desired precision, be defined as:

$$\varepsilon = |\hat{\theta} - \theta|/\theta$$

In the present example it follows that

$$|p - P| = z_{1-\alpha/2} \frac{\sqrt{P(1-P)}}{\sqrt{n}}$$

and, dividing both sides by P, we obtain an expression similar to the one presented above for ε is obtained. That is,

$$\varepsilon = \frac{|p-P|}{P} = z_{1-\alpha/2} \frac{\sqrt{(1-P)}}{\sqrt{nP}}$$

and squaring both sides and solving for n gives:

---

[e] See pages 55-57
[f] See page 86
[g] See pages 84-86

$$n = z_{1-\alpha/2}^2 \frac{(1-P)}{\varepsilon^2 P} \qquad\qquad (2)$$

Tables 2a - 2c present values of n from formula (2) for $\varepsilon = 0.01, 0.02, 0.03, 0.04, 0.05,$ 0.10, 0.15, 0.20, 0.25, 0.30, 0.35, 0.40, and 0.50, and proportions ranging from 0.05 to 0.95 in increments of 0.05. Tables are presented for 99%, 95%, and 90% confidence.

Example I.1.4
Consider the information given in Example I.1.1, only this time we will determine the sample size necessary to estimate the proportion vaccinated in the population to within 10% (*not 10 percentage points*) of the true value.

Solution
In the present example, assuming P=0.5, and using formula (2),

$$n = [(1.960)^2 \,(0.5)\,]/[\,(0.10)^2\,(0.5)\,] = 384.16.$$

Hence 385 individuals should be sampled in order to be 95% confident that the resulting estimate will fall between 0.45 and 0.55. This value can also be found in Table 2b in the column headed 0.50 and the row headed 0.10. Notice that a much larger sample size of 385 is necessary to estimate P to within 10% of the true value than that of 97 which was necessary previously to estimate P to within 10 percentage points.

Example I.1.5
How large a sample would be required to estimate the proportion of pregnant women in the population who seek prenatal care within the first trimester of pregnancy to within 5% of the true value with 95% confidence. It is estimated that the proportion of women seeking such care will be somewhere between 25% and 40%.

Solution
Using Table 2b it can be seen that if P=0.25, 4610 women would have to be sampled to estimate P to within 5% of P with 95% confidence; if P=0.30, in Table 2b shows that 3586 would be necessary; if P=0.35, n=2854; and if P were as large as 0.40, 2305 women would have to be studied. Therefore, a study might be planned with roughly n=4610 women to satisfy the objectives of the study. If, however, this number is too large then a smaller sample size might be used with a loss of either precision or confidence or both.

In the above situations, the primary aim was to estimate the population proportion. We now consider sample size determination where there is an underlying hypothesis which is to be tested.

Hypothesis testing for a single population proportion

Suppose we would like to test the hypothesis[h]

$$H_0: P = P_0$$

versus the alternative hypothesis

$$H_a: P > P_0$$

and we would like to fix the level of the type I error to equal α and the type II error to

[h] See pages 64-67

equal β. That is, we want the power of the test[i] to equal $1-\beta$. Without loss of generality, we will denote the actual P in the population as P_a. This may be represented graphically as shown in Fig. 2:

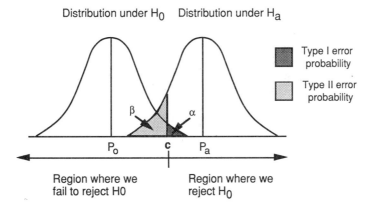

Distribution under H_0 Distribution under H_a

Type I error probability

Type II error probability

P_0 c P_a

Region where we fail to reject H0

Region where we reject H_0

Fig. 2 Sampling distributions for one-sample hypothesis test

In this figure the point "**c**" represents, for the sampling distribution centered at P_0 (i.e., the distribution which would result if the null hypothesis were true), the upper $100(\alpha)$th percent point of the distribution of p:

$$c = P_0 + z_{1-\alpha}\sqrt{[P_0(1-P_0)/n]}$$

and, for the sampling distribution centered at P_a (i.e., the distribution which would result if the alternate hypothesis were true), the lower $100(\beta)$th percent point of the distribution of p:

$$c = P_a - z_{1-\beta}\sqrt{[P_a(1-P_a)/n]}$$

In order to find n we set the two expressions equal to each other and solve for n. From this, it follows that:

$$P_0 + z_{1-\alpha}\sqrt{[P_0(1-P_0)/n]} = P_a - z_{1-\beta}\sqrt{[P_a(1-P_a)/n]}$$

or,

$$P_a - P_0 = \{z_{1-\alpha}\sqrt{[P_0(1-P_0)]} + z_{1-\beta}\sqrt{[P_a(1-P_a)]}\}/\sqrt{n}$$

The necessary sample size, for this single sample hypothesis testing situation, is therefore given by the formula:

---

[i] See pages 65-66

$$n = \frac{\left\{ z_{1-\alpha}\sqrt{P_0(1-P_0)} + z_{1-\beta}\sqrt{P_a(1-P_a)} \right\}^2}{(P_a - P_0)^2}$$ (3)

Formula (3) has been criticized for providing underestimates of the sample size necessary to achieve the stated level of power. As a result, various adjustments to this formula have been proposed in the statistical literature which adjust the sample sizes to make them achieve the stated goals for type-I and type-II errors more accurately. Tables 3a-3i present sample sizes corresponding to the uncorrected values computed using the above formula since we believe that researchers using this formula will certainly achieve close approximations to the desired goals, and that adding a level of precision to a process which relies heavily upon specifying levels of unknown parameters (e.g., P_a), would be of questionable value. (See Fleiss[18] for the modification of the sample size formula based on the continuity correction.)

Example I.1.6
During a virulent outbreak of neonatal tetanus, health workers wish to determine whether the rate is decreasing after a period during which it had risen to a level of 150 cases per thousand live births. What sample size is necessary to test $H_0:P=0.15$ at the 0.05 level if it is desired to have a 90% probability of detecting a rate of 100 per thousand if that were the true proportion?

Solution
Using formula (3), it follows that

$$n = \{1.645\sqrt{[(0.15)(0.85)]} + 1.282\sqrt{[(0.10)(0.90)]}\}^2/(0.05)^2 = 377.90.$$

So, a total sample size of 378 live births would be necessary. An alternative to performing this computation would be to look up the sample size directly in Table 3d with $P_0=0.15$, $P_a=0.10$, $\alpha=0.05$, and $\beta=0.10$ (since the desired power is 90%). In that table we find again that a sample of size 378 would be required. Notice that as P_a gets further and further away from P_0, the necessary sample size decreases.

Note that when using Tables 3a-3i, the values of P_0 and P_a are *not* interchangeable. Columns are headed by values of P_0 and rows by values of P_a. Entering the table in an inappropriate manner will result in wrong sample size determination.

Example I.1.7
Previous surveys have demonstrated that the usual rate of dental caries among school children in a particular community is about 25%. How many children should be studied in a new survey if it is desired to be 80% sure of detecting a level of 20% or less at the 0.05 level of significance?

Solution
Using Table 3e, using the row headed 0.20, and moving to the column headed 0.25, it can be seen that a sample of 441 children must be studied.

Note that in order to calculate n, α, β, P_0 and P_a must be specified. A similar approach is followed when the alternative is two-sided. That is, suppose we wish to test

$$H_0: P = P_0$$

versus

$$H_a: P \neq P_0$$

Fig. 3 presents the sampling distributions for this situation.

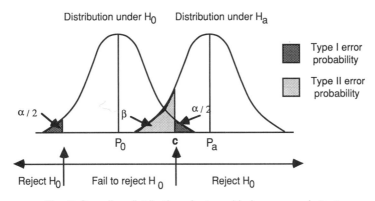

Fig. 3 Sampling distributions for two-sided, one-sample test

From this figure we see that the null hypothesis is rejected if p, the observed proportion, is too large or too small. We assign area $\alpha/2$ to each tail of the sampling distribution under H_0. The power of the test is the area under the distribution centered at P_a which falls in the rejection region. However, it should be noted that if P_a is greater than P_0, the probability of a proportion sampled from the distribution centered at P_a falling into the lower portion of the critical region of the sampling distribution centered at P_0 will be very small. On the other hand, if the picture were reversed, and P_a was smaller than P_0, then the probability of a proportion sampled from the distribution centered at P_a falling into the upper portion of the critical region of the sampling distribution centered at P_0 will be very small.

The only adjustment to the sample size formula (3) presented for the one-tailed test is that $z_{1-\alpha/2}$ will be used in place of $z_{1-\alpha}$. This can be derived by noting that "c" represents, for the sampling distribution centered at P_0 (i.e., the distribution which would result if the null hypothesis were true), the upper $100(\alpha/2)^{th}$ percent point of the distribution of p:

$$c = P_0 + z_{1-\alpha/2}\sqrt{[P_0(1-P_0)/n]}$$

and, for the sampling distribution centered at P_a (i.e., the distribution which would result if the alternate hypothesis were true), the lower $100(\beta)^{th}$ percent point:

$$c = P_a - z_{1-\beta}\sqrt{[P_a(1-P_a)/n]}$$

Then, setting the two expressions equal to each other and solving for n, it follows that:

$$n = \frac{\left\{ z_{1-\alpha/2}\sqrt{P_0(1-P_0)} + z_{1-\beta}\sqrt{P_a(1-P_a)} \right\}^2}{(P_a - P_0)^2} \tag{4}$$

In determining sample size for this one-sample, two-sided hypothesis testing situation, the problem is that we cannot be sure whether P_a was larger than or smaller than P_0. Hence, to determine adequate sample size, it is necessary to compute n twice; once with P_a larger by a stated amount than P_0 and again with P_a less than P_0 by that stated amount. The appropriate sample size is the larger of these two numbers.

Tables 4a-4i present sample sizes corresponding to formula (4) for a range of values of P_0, P_a, α and β. These tables are accessed by selecting the column corresponding to P_0 (or $1-P_0$ if $P_0 >0.5$) and the row corresponding to the absolute value of the difference between P_0 and P_a ($|P_0 - P_a|$).

Example I.1.8
Suppose the success rate for surgical treatment of a particular heart condition is widely reported in the literature to be 0.70. A new medical treatment has been proposed which is alleged to offer equivalent treatment success. A hospital without the necessary surgical facilities or staff has decided to use the new medical treatment on all new patients presenting with this condition. How many patients must be studied to test $H_0:P=0.70$ versus $H_a:P\neq0.70$ at the 0.05 level if it is desired to have 90% power of detecting a difference in proportion of success of 10 percentage points or greater?

Solution
Using formula (4) we first consider P_a greater than P_0 by 10% (i.e., $P_a =0.8$).

$$n = [1.960\sqrt{\{(0.7)(0.3)\}} + 1.282\sqrt{\{(0.8)(0.2)\}}]^2/[0.1]^2 = 199.09.$$

Hence, a total sample size of 200 patients would be necessary. Similarly, since P_a may be less than P_0 by 10 percentage points, the computations are performed again using $P_a =0.6$.

$$n = [1.960\sqrt{\{(0.7)(0.3)\}} + 1.282\sqrt{\{(0.6)(0.4)\}}]^2/[0.1]^2 = 232.94.$$

Hence, taking the larger of the two sample size determinations, we would require 233 patients to be studied using the new medical treatment. This number may be found directly by entering Table 4d in the column corresponding to $1-P_0=0.3$ and the row corresponding to $|P_0-P_a|=0.10$.

Example I.1.9
The proportion of patients seeking prenatal care in the first trimester of pregnancy is estimated to be 40% according to figures released by a local department of health. Health officials in another county are interested in comparing their success at providing prenatal care with the published data. How many women should be sampled in order to test $H_0:P=0.40$ versus $H_a:P\neq0.40$ in order to be 80% confident of detecting a difference of as much as 5 percentage points with $\alpha=0.05$?

Solution
Using formula (4) we first consider P_a to be 5 percentage points greater than P_0 (i.e., $P_a=0.45$).

$$n = [1.960\sqrt{\{(0.4)(0.6)\}} + 0.842\sqrt{\{(0.45)(0.55)\}}]^2/[0.05]^2 = 760.76.$$

Hence, a total sample size of 761 patients would be necessary. Similarly, since P_a may be less than P_0 by 5 percentage points, the computations are performed again using $P_a =0.35$.

$$n = [1.960\sqrt{\{(0.4)(0.6)\}} + 0.842\sqrt{\{(0.35)(0.65)\}}]^2/[0.05]^2 = 741.81.$$

Hence, taking the larger of the two sample size determinations, we would require 761 patients to be studied in the community. This number may be found directly by entering Table 4e in the column corresponding to $P_0=0.40$ and the row corresponding to $|P_0-P_a|=0.05$.

2 The two-sample problem

Up to now all attention has focused on the situation where a single sample has been selected from some population and we either estimated a parameter in the population or tested a hypothesis concerning it. We now focus on estimating the difference between two population proportions and on testing hypotheses concerning the equality of proportions in two groups.

Estimating the difference between two proportions

The difference between two population proportions represents a new parameter, P_1-P_2. In the epidemiologic literature, this difference is called the **risk difference**[j] and gives the absolute difference in risk between two groups. In other types of studies, the difference between the proportions may have different interpretation. An estimate of this parameter is given by the difference in the sample proportions, p_1-p_2. The mean of the sampling distribution of p_1-p_2[k] is

$$E(p_1-p_2) = P_1-P_2$$

and the variance of this distribution is

$$Var(p_1-p_2) = Var(p_1) + Var(p_2) = P_1(1-P_1)/n_1 + P_2(1-P_2)/n_2.$$

Since the values of P_1 and P_2 are unknown population parameters, replacing them with the values of p_1 and p_2 provides an estimate of the variance which can be used for the purpose of constructing a confidence interval estimate of the risk difference, P_1-P_2. That is, the upper and lower bounds on the confidence interval are given by

$$(p_1-p_2) \pm z_{1-\alpha/2} \sqrt{[p_1(1-p_1)/n_1+p_2(1-p_2)/n_2]}$$

Example I.2.1
Suppose two drugs are available for the treatment of a particular type of intestinal parasite. One hundred patients entering a clinic for treatment for this parasite are randomized to one of the two drugs; fifty receiving the standard drug A and fifty receiving drug B. Of the patients receiving drug A, 64% responded favorably; 82% of the patients receiving drug B responded favorably. Estimate the difference between the proportions responding favorably to the two drugs with a 95% confidence interval.

Solution
The end points of the 95% confidence interval estimate for the difference are as follows:

$$(p_1-p_2) \pm z_{1-\alpha/2} \sqrt{[p_1(1-p_1)/n_1+p_2(1-p_2)/n_2]}$$

$$(0.64-0.82) \pm 1.960\sqrt{[(0.64)(0.36)/50+(0.82)(0.18)/50]}$$

$$-0.18 \pm 1.960(0.0869) = -0.18 \pm 0.17.$$

The resulting 95% confidence interval for P_1-P_2 is

$$-0.35 \leq P_1-P_2 \leq -0.01.$$

The fact that zero does not fall in this interval suggests that the two drugs may

---
[j] See pages 71-78
[k] See page 57

not be equally effective in the treatment of patients with intestinal parasites.

Now suppose a study is being planned and it is desired to produce a confidence interval which can estimate the risk difference with certain precision. For example, we might want to be 95% confident of estimating the risk difference to within 2 percentage points of the true risk difference. Or we might want to estimate the risk difference to within 10% of the true difference.

$$Var(p_1-p_2) = Var(p_1) + Var(p_2) = P_1(1-P_1)/n_1 + P_2(1-P_2)/n_2.$$

If $n_1 = n_2 = n$ then

$$Var(p_1-p_2) = (1/n)\{P_1(1-P_1)+P_2(1-P_2)\}.$$

Unless we have an estimate of P_1 and P_2 (from the literature or a pilot sample), we will take the most conservative estimate possible of 0.5 for each of P_1 and P_2 should be used. Then,

$$Var(p_1-p_2) = (1/n)\{(0.5)(0.5)+(0.5)(0.5)\} = (1/n)(0.5) = 1/2n.$$

Now, following the same logic as was used in estimating a single population proportion, the quantity d denotes the distance, in either direction, from the population risk difference and may be expressed as

$$d = z_{1-\alpha/2}\sqrt{[(1/n)\{P_1(1-P_1)+P_2(1-P_2)\}]}.$$

Solving this expression for n it follows that

$$n = \frac{z_{1-\alpha/2}^2[P_1(1-P_1) + P_2(1-P_2)]}{d^2} \qquad (5)$$

When it is desired that n_2 be proportionate to n_1 (i.e., $n_2=kn_1$) then expression (5) transforms to:

$$n = \frac{z_{1-\alpha/2}^2[kP_1(1-P_1) + P_2(1-P_2)]}{kd^2}$$

Tables are provided for determining the sample size of formula (5) in a two-stage process. First Table 5a is used to obtain the value of "V" given by:

$$P_1(1-P_1) + P_2(1-P_2)$$

(P_1 and P_2 may be interchanged for the purpose of obtaining the value of V from this table. When P_1 and P_2 are unknown, the table is entered at $P_1 = 0.5$, and $P_2 = 0.5$ which yields the value of $V = 0.5$.) Then once V has been determined from Table 5a, we determine the required sample size using Table 5b, 5c, or 5d (corresponding to $\alpha=0.01$, 0.05 and 0.10, respectively), by looking up the intersection of the row corresponding to V and the column corresponding to d%. When the precise values cannot be located in these tables, estimates may be obtained by interpolation.

Example I.2.2
If it is desired to estimate a risk difference to an environmental exposure in two industrial groups, how large a sample should be selected in each group for the estimate to be within 5 percentage points of the true difference with 95% confidence, when no reasonable estimates of exposure risks for either group are available?

Solution
Here d=0.05, so using formula (5), it follows that

$$n = 1.960^2[0.5(0.5)+0.5(0.5)]/(0.05)^2 = 768.32.$$

Hence, a study with 769 subjects in each of two groups would be required. This same value may be found in the tables by first looking up V in Table 5a, ($P_1=P_2=0.50$, so V=0.50) and then going to the column corresponding to d%=5 in Table 5c, and the row corresponding to V=0.5.

Example I.2.3
Suppose that in a pilot study using 50 patients in each of two groups it was observed that $p_1=0.40$ and $p_2=0.32$. The estimated risk difference is p_1-p_2 = 0.08. If we would like to estimate the population risk difference to within 5 percentage points of the true value with 95% confidence, how many additional patients must be studied?

Solution
Using the sample proportions as estimates of the population parameters it follows that

$$n = 1.960^2 [(0.40)(0.60)+(0.32)(0.68)]/(0.05)^2 = 703.17.$$

Hence, 704 patients would be required in each of the two groups. Since 50 were enrolled in each group for the pilot study, 656 *additional* patients must be studied in each group. Note that by using the pilot data, we were able to reduce the sample size estimates produced in the previous example where the conservative variance estimate was used. This value may be looked up directly by using , first, Table 5a which gives a value of V of 0.46 and then Table 5c in the row headed by 0.46 and the column headed by 5 for the sample size value of 707. (The discrepancy between 707 using Table 5c and 704 as computed using formula (5) results from the fact that V is actually equal to 0.4576 rather than the 0.46 given in Table 5a. For purposes of sample size determination, errors of this size are unimportant.)

By defining $\theta = P_1-P_2$, it is possible to derive an expression to estimate the risk difference to within ε of the true value, similar to that done in the one sample case. However, it is our impression that for risk difference, a fixed precision will usually be stated in terms of the value previously denoted by "d". Therefore, this alternative parametrization is not discussed further in this manual.

Hypothesis testing for two population proportions

Suppose a study is designed to test[1] H_0: $P_1=P_2$ versus H_a: $P_1>P_2$. The mean of the sampling distribution of p_1-p_2 under H_0 is 0 and the variance is

$$Var(p_1-p_2) = Var(p_1) +Var(p_2) = P_1(1-P_1)/n_1 + P_2(1-P_2)/n_2 .$$

If we let the hypothesized common value of P_1 and P_2 be denoted by P, then

$$Var(p_1-p_2) = P(1-P)/n_1 + P(1-P)/n_2 = P(1-P)(1/n_1+1/n_2)$$

and if $n_1=n_2=n$, then

$$Var(p_1-p_2) = 2[P(1-P)/n] .$$

Clearly, this variance involves the population parameter, P, which we have no way of

---

[1] See pages 64-67

knowing. This parameter may be estimated as the average of the two-sample proportions from the pilot study. That is,

$$\hat{P} = \bar{p} = (p_1 + p_2)/2 .$$

Fig 4 displays a graphical representation of the two sample hypothesis testing situation for two proportions.

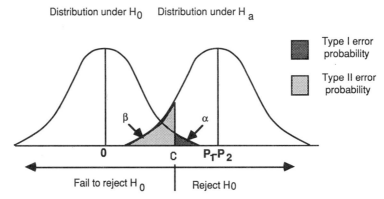

Distribution under H_0 Distribution under H_a

Type I error probability

Type II error probability

β α

0   c P_T-P_2

Fail to reject H_0 | Reject H_0

Fig. 4 Two-sample, one-sided test of $H_0 : P_1 = P_2$ vs $H_a: P_1 > P_2$

Example I.2.4
Consider the data of Example I.2.1. One hundred patients entered a clinic for treatment of a particular parasite and participated in a randomized trial of the two drugs; fifty received drug A which is the standard treatment and fifty received a new drug, drug B. This new drug will be adopted if it can be demonstrated, at the $\alpha = 0.05$ level, that it is more effective than the standard treatment. Of the patients receiving drug A, 64% responded favorably; 82% of the patients receiving drug B responded favorably. Is drug B significantly more effective than drug A? In other words, is the observed difference too large to be due to chance alone?

Solution
Using $\alpha = 0.05$, the decision rule is to reject H_0 if $p_1 - p_2$ is greater than $0 + 1.64\sqrt{2(0.73)(0.27)/50} = 0.146$. The value 0.73 is the average of the proportions responding in each group (previously denoted $\bar{p}$). In the actual trial, letting p_1 and p_2 denote the proportion with a favorable response with drugs B and A respectively, $p_1 - p_2 = 0.82 - 0.64 = 0.18$. Therefore, since this falls in the rejection region, the null hypothesis is rejected in favor of the alternative that drug B is more effective than drug A.

Now, suppose we would like to consider the previously described trial as a pilot study, and assuming that a difference in proportions of 0.18 is considered clinically significant, how many patients should be studied in order to be 90% confident of rejecting H_0 when, in fact the true difference between the population proportions is 0.18?

As is seen in Fig. 4, under H_0 the point c is defined as

$$c = z_{1-\alpha}\sqrt{[2\bar{P}(1-\bar{P})/n]},$$

where $\bar{P} = (P_1+P_2)/2$. Under H_a,

$$c = (P_1-P_2) - z_{1-\beta}\sqrt{[P_1(1-P_1)/n_1+P_2(1-P_2)/n_2]}$$

and, assuming $n_1=n_2=n$, equating these equations and solving for n we obtain

$$n = \frac{\left\{z_{1-\alpha}\sqrt{2\bar{P}(1-\bar{P})} + z_{1-\beta}\sqrt{P_1(1-P_1)+P_2(1-P_2)}\right\}^2}{(P_1-P_2)^2} \qquad (6)$$

Tables 6a-6i give, for various choices of α and β, the sample sizes of formula (6).

Example I.2.5
Suppose it has been estimated that the rate of caries is 800 per 1000 school children in one district and 600 per 1000 in another district. How large a sample of children from each district is required to determine whether this difference is significant at the 10% level if we wish to have an 80% chance of detecting the difference if it is real?

Solution
Using formula (6) with $\bar{P} = (0.80+0.60)/2=0.70$, it follows that

$$n = \{1.282\sqrt{[2(0.70)(0.30)]}+0.842\sqrt{[(0.80)(0.20)+(0.60)(0.40)]}\}^2/(0.80-0.60)^2$$

$$= 46.47.$$

Hence, a sample of 47 children from *each* district would be required.   Using Table 6h it can be seen from the intersection of the column headed 0.60 and the row headed 0.80 that $n = 47$.

A similar approach is followed when the alternative is two-sided.   That is, suppose we wish to test $H_0:P_1-P_2=0$ versus $H_a:P_1-P_2\neq0$. Fig. 5 presents the sampling distributions for this situation.

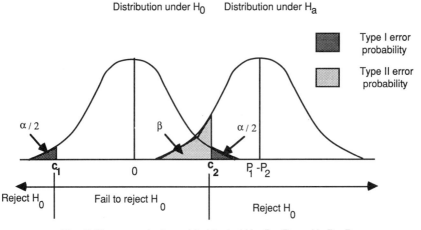

Fig. 5 Two-sample, two-sided test of $H_0: P_1=P_2$ vs $H_a:P_1\neq P_2$

Note that H_0 is rejected if $p_1-p_2 > c_2$ or if $p_1-p_2 < c_1$. If H_0 is false, and if $P_1-P_2 > 0$, it will be a very rare event for p_1-p_2 to be less than c_1. With that in mind, note that c_2 may be defined with respect to either distribution. For the distribution centered at 0,

$$c_2 = 0 + z_{1-\alpha/2}\sqrt{[2\bar{P}(1-\bar{P})/n]}$$

and, for the sampling distribution centered at P_1-P_2 (i.e., the distribution which would result if the alternative hypothesis were true):

$$c_2 = P_1-P_2 - z_{1-\beta}\sqrt{[P_1(1-P_1)/n+P_2(1-P_2)/n]} .$$

Then, setting the two expressions equal to each other and solving for n it follows that

$$n = \frac{\left\{ z_{1-\alpha/2}\sqrt{2\bar{P}(1-\bar{P})} + z_{1-\beta}\sqrt{P_1(1-P_1) + P_2(1-P_2)} \right\}^2}{(P_1-P_2)^2} \tag{7}$$

Tables 7a-7i present, for various choices of α and β, the sample sizes based on formula (7). The necessary sample size is found at the intersection of the column corresponding to the smaller of P_1 and P_2, and if neither of these proportions is less than 0.5, then the smaller of $1-P_1$ and $1-P_2$ is used as the column in which to enter the table. The appropriate row corresponds to the absolute value of the difference between P_1 and P_2, i.e., $|P_1-P_2|$.

Example I.2.6
An epidemiologist compared, in a pilot survey, a sample of 50 adult subjects suffering from a certain neurologic disease to a sample of 50 comparable control subjects who were free of the disease. Thirty of the subjects with the disease (60%) and 25 of the controls (50%) were involved in industries using a specific chemical. Assuming that the proportion employed in these industries in the entire population is similar to that observed in the pilot survey, how many additional subjects should be studied in each of the two groups to have 90% confidence of detecting the true difference between the groups if the hypothesis is tested at the 5% level?

Solution
Using formula (7), assuming P_1=0.60, P_2=0.50, α=0.05, and β=0.10, it follows that

$$n = \{1.960\sqrt{[2(0.55)(0.45)]} + 1.282\sqrt{[0.6(0.4)+0.5(0.5)]}\}^2/(0.6-0.5)^2 = 518.19.$$

Hence, a sample size of 519 subjects is required in each of the two groups. Since 50 were already chosen in the pilot survey, an additional 469 subjects are required in each group. This same result may be obtained using Table 7d., where it can be seen from the intersection of the column headed 0.40 and the row headed 0.10, that n=519.

It should be noted that the above method is just an approximation since several distributional assumptions were made. Fleiss[18] presents tables for sample size in the two-group problem for a two-sided alternative. These tables are based upon an adjustment originally proposed by Casagrande, Pike and Smith[6] which modifies the sample size as given by formula (7) in the following manner:

$$n' = (n/4)(1+\sqrt{[1+4/\{n|P_2-P_1|\}]}).$$

In the situation where the underlying rate is very rare (e.g. in a disease such as cancer having an underlying probability of occurrence of 50 per 100,000 or 0.0005), neither of the above methods may be appropriate. Lemeshow, Hosmer and Stewart[41] demonstrated that for diseases whose occurrence is rare, the arcsin formula performed best. That is,

$$n = \frac{(z_{1-\alpha} + z_{1-\beta})^2}{2\left(\arcsin\sqrt{P_2} - \arcsin\sqrt{P_1} \right)^2}$$ (8)

Sample sizes based on formula (8) are given in Tables 8a-8i for various choices of α, β, P_1 and P_2.

Example I.2.7
Two communities are to be identified to participate in a study to evaluate widescale use of a new screening program for early identification of a particular type of cancer. In one community, the screening program will be used on all adults over the age of 35, while in the second community it will not be used at all. The annual incidence rate of this type of cancer is 50/100,000=0.0005 in an unscreened population. A drop in the rate to 20/100,000=0.0002 would justify using the procedure on a widespread basis. How many adults should be followed in each of the two communities to have an 80% probability of detecting a drop in the rate this large if the hypothesis test will be performed at the 5% level of significance?

Solution
Using formula (8):

$$n = (1.645+0.84)^2/\{2(\arcsin\sqrt{0.0005} - \arcsin\sqrt{0.0002})^2\}$$
$$= (1.645+0.84)^2/\{2(0.0223625432 - 0.014142607)^2\}$$
$$= 45770.39$$

Hence, 45771 adults should be studied in each community. Alternatively, looking up Table 8e, from the intersection of the column P_1=0.0002 and the row P_2=0.0005, it can be seen that the required sample size is 45771.

3 Sample size for case-control studies

Estimating the odds ratio[m] with stated precision ε

With some simple modifications, the solution to this problem follows directly from the results developed earlier about estimation of any unknown parameter θ. Because the odds ratio (OR) is strictly positive and since, in practice, the odds ratio is rarely larger than 10 and usually much smaller, it follows that the sampling distribution of the estimated odds ratio will tend to be nonnormal (except for extremely large samples) with strong positive skewness. In cases such as this, the natural logarithm ($\log_e$ denoted by "ln") transformation will often improve the distributional properties. That is, the sampling distribution of ln(OR) will be more nearly normally distributed than that of OR for any given sample size. As a result, the most commonly employed large-sample method for determining a confidence interval estimate for the odds ratio, or for testing hypotheses about the odds ratio, is based on ln(OR). For confidence intervals, once the end points have been determined on a logarithmic scale they may be transformed to the original scale by exponentiation. That is,

$$e^{\ln(OR)} = OR .$$

Following exponentiation of the end points, the resulting confidence interval will be asymmetric, the direction of the skew depending upon whether the end points of the confidence interval for ln(OR) are greater or less than one.

For a case-control study denoting the probabilities of exposure given disease presence or absence by P_1^* and P_2^* respectively, the variance of the sampling distribution of ln(OR), for $n_1 = n_2 = n$, is approximated as:

$$Var[\ln(O\hat{R})] \cong 1/[nP_1^*] + 1/[n(1-P_1^*)] + 1/[nP_2^*] + 1/[n(1-P_2^*)] .$$

Since this expression involves unknown population parameters, an estimate of this quantity may be obtained from a pilot survey, or other data sources, as[n]:

$$Var[\ln(O\hat{R})] = 1/a + 1/b + 1/c + 1/d ,$$

where the values a, b, c, and d are obtained from a 2x2 cross tabulation as shown in Table I.1.

If a test of H_0:OR=1 versus against the alternative H_a:OR≠1 is to be performed, the usual test is based on the chi-square (χ^2) test computed from the 2x2 table. If the resulting calculated value of χ^2 is too large (i.e., $\chi^2 > \chi^2_{1-\alpha}$(1 degree of freedom)), the null hypothesis is rejected.

We would like to know what sample size, n, is necessary to estimate the OR to within ε of OR with probability 1-α. Fig. 6 depicts the use of the ln(OR) and the relationship between the end points of the confidence intervals as defined on two scales.

---

[m] See pages 71-78
[n] See pages 74-75

Table I.1 Tabular display of disease/exposure relationship

	Exposure		
Disease	Present (E)	Absent (Ē)	Total
Present (D)	a	b	n_1
Absent (D̄)	c	d	n_2
Total	m_1	m_2	n

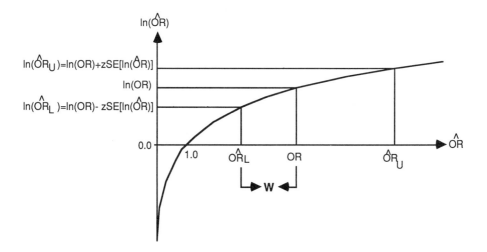

Fig. 6 Plot of confidence interval for ln(OR) vs. confidence interval for OR

We know that, based on the log scale, with 100(1-α)% confidence, the value of ln(OR) falls somewhere between ln($\hat{OR}_U$) and ln($\hat{OR}_L$) in Fig. 6. Note that whereas the interval established for ln(OR) is symmetric, when the values are exponentiated they yield an asymmetric interval on the OR scale.

We wish to determine the number of study subjects, n, required in each of the case and control groups so that the width of the stated portion of the interval be of length w, with probability 1-α.

A number of assumptions are made at this point. First we assume that the OR > 1. If this is not the case, the reader may proceed simply by interchanging the definition of "exposed" and "unexposed". Second, we wish to control the width of the left half of the confidence interval ("w" in Fig. 6) since controlling the distance between OR_U and OR would usually result in unrealistically large sample size requirements. It will be useful to define the width w as a function of the odds ratio so we choose n to estimate the OR to within ε of its true value. We do this via the equation w=εOR, where ε=| $\hat{OR}_L$-OR|/OR. It follows from Fig. 6 that

$$w = \varepsilon OR = e^{\ln(OR)} - e^{\ln(OR) - zSE(\ln(OR))}$$
$$\varepsilon OR = OR - ORe^{-zSE(\ln(OR))}$$
$$\varepsilon = 1 - e^{-zSE(\ln(OR))}$$
$$1 - \varepsilon = e^{-zSE(\ln(OR))}$$
$$\ln(1-\varepsilon) = -z_{1-\alpha/2} SE(\ln(OR))$$
$$\ln(1-\varepsilon) = -z_{1-\alpha/2} \sqrt{[(1/n)\{1/[P_1^*(1-P_1^*)] + 1/[P_2^*(1-P_2^*)]\}]}$$

and solving for n,

$$n = \frac{z_{1-\alpha/2}^2 \{1/[P_1^*(1-P_1^*)] + 1/[P_2^*(1-P_2^*)]\}}{[\ln(1-\varepsilon)]^2} \qquad (9)$$

Note that in solving these problems there are three parameters (P_1^*, P_2^* and OR) but only two need be specified since any two determine the third. For example, if P_2^* and OR are given then

$$P_1^* = \frac{(OR) P_2^*}{(OR) P_2^* + (1 - P_2^*)}$$

Tables 9a-9l present the sample sizes for 99%, 95%, and 90% confidence intervals, ε = 0.10, 0.20, 0.25 and 0.50, odds ratios ranging from 1.25 to 4.0 and P_2^* ranging from 0.01 to 0.90.

Example I.3.1
What sample size would be needed in each of two groups for a case-control study to be 95% confident of estimating the population odds ratio to within 25% of the true value if this true value is believed to be in the vicinity of 2, and the exposure rate among the controls is estimated to be 0.30?

Solution
The proportion exposed among the cases is

$$P_1^* = OR \cdot P_2^* / [OR \cdot P_2^* + (1-P_2^*)]$$

$$= 2 \times 0.3 / [2 \times 0.3 + 0.7] = 0.46$$

Evaluating the required sample size from formula (9) it follows that

$$n = (1.960)^2 [1/\{0.46 \times 0.54\} + 1/\{0.3 \times 0.7\}]/[\ln(1-0.25)]^2 = 407.91.$$

Hence, 408 subjects would be required in each of the case and control groups in order to assure, with 95% confidence, that the estimate of the odds ratio will not underestimate the true OR by more than 25% of its true value. Using Table 9g the same result is obtained. The table is entered in the column for OR=2.00 and the row for P_2^*=0.30. At the intersection of this row and column it can be seen that n=408.

Example I.3.2
If, in Example I.3.1, we want the estimate to be within 50% of the true odds ratio, what should be the minimum sample size for each study group?

Solution
The calculations for sample size in this example are as follows:

$$n = (1.960)^2 [1/\{0.46 \times 0.54\} + 1/\{0.3 \times 0.7\}]/[\ln(1-0.5)]^2 = 70.26.$$

Hence, only 71 subjects would be required in each of the two groups. This value may be looked up directly in Table 9h.

The above example demonstrates an important point relevant to sample size for estimating the population odds ratio. Specifically, estimation of the odds ratio with a level of precision commonly used with such other population parameters as proportions or means, requires very large samples. (Had we required the estimate to be within 10% of the true value, a sample size of 3041 would have been required in each group.)

Sample size for hypothesis testing of the odds ratio

If the goal of the statistical analysis is to test a hypothesis about the odds ratio, the sample size calculations may be performed using previously described methodology. The only additional step required is to translate the alternative hypothesis from one which involves the odds ratio to an equivalent statement about proportions.

When testing hypotheses about the odds ratio, the most common null hypothesis is that of no effect due to the exposure variable. Under the null hypothesis the odds ratio is 1, i.e., H_0: OR=1, and the proportion exposed among the cases is equal to the proportion exposed among the controls. Thus, the null hypothesis is equivalent to that of equality of two proportions. For a specified alternative hypothesis that the odds ratio is some number different from 1, i.e. OR $\neq$ 1, the proportion exposed in the cases is given by

$$P_1^* = \frac{(OR)\,P_2^*}{(OR)\,P_2^* + (1 - P_2^*)}$$

and the null and alternative hypotheses expressed in terms of proportions are

$$H_0: P_1^* = P_2^*$$

versus

$$H_a: P_1^* \neq P_2^*$$

where P_1^* is given above and P_2^* is known.

The sample size needed to test these null and alternative hypotheses has already been presented in the discussion of two-sample hypothesis testing of proportions. The formula, similar to formula (7), is repeated below with minor modifications.

$$n = \frac{\left\{ z_{1-\alpha/2}\sqrt{2P_2^*(1 - P_2^*)} + z_{1-\beta}\sqrt{P_1^*(1 - P_1^*) + P_2^*(1 - P_2^*)} \right\}^2}{(P_1^* - P_2^*)^2} \tag{10}$$

Note that in the above formula we have used $2P_2^*(1-P_2^*)$ in place of $2\,\bar{P}^*(1-\bar{P}^*)$ as was used previously (where $\bar{P}^* = (P_1^* + P_2^*)/2$). The rationale for this modification is that it is likely that the population is made up of many more individuals without the condition (controls) than it is of individuals with the condition (cases). Often the exposure rate among the controls will be known with a high degree of precision and, under the null hypothesis, this is the exposure rate for the cases as well. Thus it seems logical to use P_2^* as the population proportion for each group. The use of $2\bar{P}(1-\bar{P})$ in the formula in the earlier development was to provide a method of expressing uncertainty with respect to the common proportion of the two groups. If one is not sure of the exposure rate among the controls then one should use $2\,\bar{P}^*(1-\bar{P}^*)$ with formula (10).

Tables 10a-10i present sample sizes corresponding to formula (10). The table is accessed by specifying α (0.01, 0.05 or 0.10), β (0.10, 0.20 or 0.50), OR (ranging from 0.25 to 4.00) and P_2^* (ranging from 0.01 to 0.90).

The following example will illustrate the use of P_2^* versus $\bar{P}^*$.

Example I.3.3
The efficacy of BCG vaccine in preventing childhood tuberculosis is in doubt and a study is designed to compare the immunization coverage rates in a group of tuberculosis cases compared to a group of controls. Available information indicates that roughly 30% of the controls are not vaccinated, and we wish to have an 80% chance of detecting whether the odds ratio is significantly different from 1 at the 5% level. If an odds ratio of 2 would be considered an important difference between the two groups, how large a sample should be included in each study group?

Solution
The exposure rate (proportion unvaccinated) among the cases which yields an odds ratio of 2 is

$$P_1^* = 2 \times 0.3/[2 \times 0.3 + 0.7] = 0.4615$$

Now, using formula (10), it follows that

$$n = \frac{\left[1.960 \sqrt{2 \times 0.3 \times 0.7} + 0.842 \sqrt{0.4615 \times 0.5385 + 0.3 \times 0.7} \right]^2}{(0.4615 - 0.3)^2}$$

$$= 129.79$$

Thus 130 cases and 130 controls would be necessary. This value may be found in Table 10e at the intersection of the column headed 2.00 and the row headed 0.30. The sample size obtained using $\bar{P}^* = [0.3 + 0.46]/2 = 0.38$ is as follows:

$$n = \frac{\left[1.960 \sqrt{2 \times 0.38 \times 0.62} + 0.842 \sqrt{0.4615 \times 0.5385 + 0.3 \times 0.7} \right]^2}{(0.4615 - 0.3)^2}$$

$$= 140.69$$

Hence 141 cases and 141 controls would be required. Which of these two sample size formulae would be used depends upon how firmly it is believed that the rate of nonvaccination among the controls, which is by far the larger group in the population, is actually 0.3.

4 Sample size determination for cohort studies

Confidence interval estimation of the relative risk

In the estimation problem we wish to estimate the relative risk[o] (RR) to within ε of the true population value. Thus, the necessary precision must first be derived using the natural logarithm (ln) scale as shown in   Fig. 7.

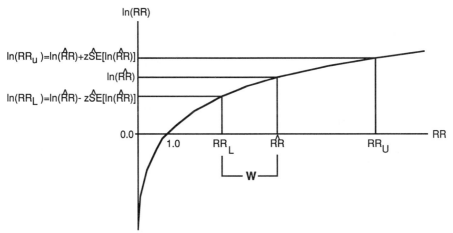

Fig.7 Plot of confidence interval for ln(RR) vs. confidence interval for RR

In this situation it follows that that

$$w = \varepsilon \cdot RR = e^{\ln(RR)} - e^{\ln(RR)-zSE(\ln(RR))}$$
$$\varepsilon \cdot RR = RR[1 - e^{-zSE[\ln(RR)]}]$$
$$1 - \varepsilon = e^{-zSE[\ln(RR)]}$$
$$\ln(1-\varepsilon) = -zSE[\ln(RR)]$$
$$\ln(1-\varepsilon) = -z\sqrt{[(1/m)\{(1-P_1)/P_1 + (1-P_2)/P_2\}]}.$$

Thus the necessary sample size is

$$m = \frac{z^2_{1-\alpha/2}[(1-P_1)/P_1 + (1-P_2)/P_2]}{[\ln(1-\varepsilon)]^2} \qquad (11)$$

Tables 11a-11l present these sample sizes for 99%, 95%, and 90% confidence intervals, $\varepsilon = 0.10, 0.20, 0.25$, and 0.50; RR ranging from 0.025 to 4.0, and P_2^* ranging from 0.01 to 0.90.

Example I.4.1
Suppose an outcome is present in 20% of the unexposed group of a cohort study, how large a sample would be needed in each of the exposed and unexposed study groups to estimate the relative risk to within 10% of the true value, which is believed to be approximately 1.75, with 95% confidence?

---

[o] See pages 71-74

Solution
It follows from the given information that

$$P_2 = 0.2$$

$$P_1 = (RR) P_2 = 0.35$$

and

$$m = (1.960)^2[(0.65/0.35) + (0.8/0.2)]/[\ln(1-0.1)]^2 = 2026.95$$

Hence a sample size of 2027 would be needed in each of the two exposure groups. This value may be located in Table 11e at the intersection of the column corresponding to RR=1.75 and the row corresponding to $P_2^* =0.20$.

Hypothesis testing of the population relative risk

The usual null hypothesis when the relative risk is the parameter of interest is H_0: RR=1. That is, it is hypothesized that the proportion of those who develop the disease is the same for both the exposed and unexposed groups. The null hypothesis may be stated equivalently in terms of these probabilities as H_0: $P_1 = P_2$. Hence, this null hypothesis is equivalent to the general null hypothesis of the equality of two proportions described earlier in Chapter 1. The alternative hypothesis may be either one or two-sided, H_a: RR>1, H_a: RR<1, or H_a: RR≠1. In each case, these may be stated equivalently in terms of the respective disease probabilities for the two groups as H_a: $P_1>P_2$, H_a: $P_1<P_2$, or H_a: $P_1≠P_2$. Thus determination of the sample size necessary to test the null hypothesis that RR=1 is fully equivalent to that for the two sample test of proportions. In most cases the quantities RR and P_2 would be specified and $P_1=RR·P_2$ would be derived.

The necessary sample size for a two-sided test would be obtained from the formula

$$n = \frac{\left\{ z_{1-\alpha/2}\sqrt{2\,p(1-p)} + z_{1-\beta}\sqrt{p_1(1-p_1) + p_2(1-p_2)} \right\}^2}{(p_1-p_2)^2} \quad (12)$$

where $p = (p_1+p_2)/2 = p_2(RR+1)/2$. Note that once p_2 is specified the value of RR is bounded by

$$0 < RR < 1/p_2 .$$

This inequality places constraints on what sample sizes are possible for a given value of p_2.

Suppose, for example, it is thought that approximately 30% of all unexposed persons may be expected to develop the disease during the time frame of the study. Then the possible values for RR are contained in the interval

$$0<RR<(1/0.3)=3.3 .$$

Hence, the alternative of H_a:RR=4 does not make sense. This is to be contrasted with the case control study where it is possible to have any value for the odds ratio for a given exposure probability for the control group. The resulting calculation for the second population given an OR and P_1^* guarantees that $0<P_2^*<1$ for any OR.

Tables 12a-12i present sample sizes based on formula (12). The tables are accessed by specifying α (0.01, 0.05, or 0.10), β (0.10, 0.20, or 0.50), RR (ranging from 0.25 to 4.00) and P_2 (ranging from 0.01 to 0.90).

Example I.4.2

Two competing therapies for a particular cancer are to be evaluated by the cohort study strategy in a multi-center clinical trial. Patients are randomized to either treatment A or B and are followed for recurrence of disease for 5 years following treatment. How many patients should be studied in each of the two arms of the trial in order to be 90% confident of rejecting H_0: RR=1 in favor of the alternative H_a:RR$\neq$1, if the test is to be performed at the α=0.05 level and if it is assumed that p_2=0.35 and RR=0.5.

Solution

Prior to using formula (12), we must compute several values. Here, RR=0.5, and p_2=0.35. Hence, $p_1 = (RR)p_2 = (0.5)(0.35) = 0.175$. Also, $p = (0.175+0.35)/2 = 0.2625$.

Now, using these values in formula (12) it follows that:

$$n = \frac{\{1.960\sqrt{[2(0.2625)(0.7375)]}+1.282\sqrt{[(0.175)(0.825)+(0.35)(0.65)]}\}^2}{(0.175-0.35)^2}$$

$$= 130.79$$

This suggests that the study be performed with 131 patients in each arm of the trial. This same sample size value may be found in Table 12d at the intersection of the column corresponding to RR=0.5 and the row corresponding to p_2=0.35.

5 Lot quality assurance sampling

The goal of health workers employing lot quality assurance sampling (LQAS) procedures is to ascertain whether or not a population meets certain standards of, for example, a health care delivery program.

The origin of these methods is in sampling and inspecting batches of a manufactured product. The strategy and goals of LQAS in the health field are similar to those in the manufacturing field. The purchaser of the goods does not want to accept a batch with more than a certain percentage (P_1) defective; the manufacturer does not want to reject the batch unless a certain percentage (P_2) are defective; it may be that $P_1 \neq P_2$. (In order to provide a health-related framework an immunization program will be used to illustrate LQAS.)

To control the more serious error of judging the population to be adequately covered ("accept the lot") when in fact it is not, the judgement procedure is set up as a one-sided test. Let "d" denote the number of persons not immunized out of a sample of "n" subjects. Let "P" denote the true proportion of individuals not immunized in the population of size "N". We will assume, as is usually the case, that N is very large relative to n. (If it happens that N is not large relative to n then the reader should consult a text such as Brownlee[3] (Sec. 3.15) which demonstrates how the hypergeometric distribution is used to evaluate the LQAS procedure.)

The null hypothesis is

$$H_0: P \geq P_0 \text{ (i.e., proportion of nonimmunized children not less than } P_0)$$

versus

$$H_a: P < P_0 \text{ (i.e., proportion of nonimmunized children less than } P_0).$$

The four-celled table presented in Fig. 8 describes the consequences of the testing procedure.

Actual Population

		Not adequately vaccinated	Adequately vaccinated	
Decision	Fail to reject H_0 "not adequate" coverage"	(test recognizes or is sensitive to lack of adequate coverage) $1-\alpha$ **sensitivity**	β **false positive rate**	"reject" the lot
	Reject H_0 "adequate" coverage"	α **false negative rate**	(test recognizes adequate coverage) $1-\beta$ **specificity**	"accept" the lot

Fig. 8 Consequences of hypothesis testing in LQAS procedure

Note that in Fig. 8, because the test is set up as one-sided, and because it is assumed the population is not adequately covered unless H_0 is rejected, the type I error, i.e., accepting the lot when it is defective (false negative), whose probability can be controlled, is the most serious error. That is, the "cost" of declaring that the population is adequately immunized, when in fact it is not, is concidered to be very high. On the other hand, the type II error, rejection of an acceptable lot, is judged not to be as serious since the result of this false-positive decision would be to take steps to improve on the immunization coverage of an already adequately immunized population.

The fundamental problem in LQAS sampling is not so much one of simply determining sample size, but of choosing an appropriate balance between sample size and critical region. The computation of β will, in all cases, depend upon what the correct value of P is when it is assumed to be different from P_0. Because LQAS surveys often use small samples, evaluation of the procedure is accomplished using the **binomial distribution.** The binomial distribution is the statistical distribution which describes the probability of a particular configuration of dichotomous outcomes when the total number is finite (e.g., the number of times a "head" appears in 7 tosses of a coin"). If P denotes the probability of observing an event, then the probability of having exactly d individuals with the event in a sample of size n is given by :

$$Prob(d) = [{}^nC_d] \, P^d \, (1-P)^{n-d} ,$$

where ${}^nC_d = n!/[d!(n-d)!]$, $a! = a \cdot (a-1) \cdot (a-2) \cdots 2 \cdot 1$ and, by definition, $0! = 1$. Thus, if 50% of the children under 2 years of age in a particular community are not immunized, the chance that we would find only 1 child who is not immunized in a random sample of 7 children in the community is:

$$Prob(1) = [{}^7C_1] \, (0.5)^1 \, (1-0.5)^6 = 0.0547 .$$

Similarly, the chance of finding exactly 1 nonimmunized child in a sample of 7 children if 70% of the children are not immunized is:

$$Prob(1) = [{}^7C_1] \, (0.7)^1 \, (1-0.7)^6 = 0.0036 .$$

Suppose we decide that 7 is the sample size we wish to use. The rejection region for the test states that we should reject H_0 (and "accept the lot" as adequately immunized) if $d \leq d^*$ (i.e., if the number of subjects in the sample found to be nonimmunized is less than or equal to the critical value, d^*). We first consider whether there is a value of d^* such that the probability that $d \leq d^*$ when H_0 is true is exactly equal to $\alpha=0.05$. The probability of $d \leq d^*$, for a specified sample size n, probability P_0, and number d^* is given by the expression

$$Prob\{d \leq d^*\} = \sum_{d=0}^{d^*} Prob(d) = \sum_{d=0}^{d^*} [{}^nC_d] \, (P_0)^d \, (1-P_0)^{n-d} \qquad (13)$$

To establish the existence of a d^* such that $Prob(d \leq d^*)=\alpha$, we must compute $Prob(d \leq d^*)$ for a number of values of d^*. In the example where n=7 and P=0.5, these values are presented in Fig. 9:

	d^*							
	0	1	2	3	4	5	6	7
$Prob\{d \leq d^*\}$	0.0078	0.0625	0.2266	0.5000	0.7734	0.9375	0.9922	1.0000

Fig. 9 Actual probability of a type I error for possible values of d^*, n=7, P=0.5

From Fig. 9 it can be seen that choosing $d^*=0$ would yield an $\alpha = 0.0078$ level test and choosing $d^*=1$ would yield an $\alpha=0.0625$ level test. If it was decided to take $n=7$ subjects, then choosing $d^*=1$ would probably be safe; but only $d^*=0$ results in a value of α less than or equal to 0.05. That is, in a sample of 7 children, none must be nonimmunized in order for us to reject H_0, thereby accepting the lot as having an immunization rate of at least 50%.

Now, if we decide to use $d^*=1$ ($\alpha=0.0625$), what is the power of the test if 70% of the population is actually nonimmunized? The probability of rejecting H_0 (i.e., accepting the lot or declaring it to have an acceptable vaccination level) is the chance that $d \leq d^*=1$, given $P=0.7$, and is computed as follows:

$$\text{Prob}\{d \leq 1\} = \sum_{d=0}^{1} [^7C_d](0.7)^d (1-0.7)^{7-d} = 0.0039 .$$

For each value of n there will be only one value of d^* at or about the chosen value of α. It is not usually possible to attain the level α exactly. Thus one choice for d^* will have the type I error less than α and d^*+1 will have type I error greater than α. The investigator will usually choose the value of d^* yielding the type I error less than α. Sometimes this strategy results in an extremely conservative test such as the one illustrated in the example above where, with $n=7$, $d^*=0$ and $P_0=0.5$, α equalled 0.0078. Here the use of $d^*=1$ with $\alpha=0.0625$ might seem justified. Tables 13a-13o give sample sizes such that α will not exceed the stated type I error probability of 0.01, 0.05 or 0.10 for various populations ($100 - \infty$), d^* ($0 - 4$) and P_0 ($0.8 - 0.1$).

Example I.5.1
Given a population of size 15000 what is the minimum sample size which should be taken so that if no more that 2 cases of malnourished children are found in the sample we can confidently say (with a probability of 95%) that the prevalence of malnutrition in the population is not more than 10%?

Solution
The general solution is to determine the value of n for which the probability of finding 2 cases in a *randomly* selected sample of size n given a population of size 15000, with 1500 malnourished children, is less than 0.05.

This probability is given by the solution of the following inequality:

$$\sum_{x=0}^{2} [^{1500}C_x \; ^{13500}C_{(n-x)}]/[^{15000}C_n] < 0.05$$

This gives $n = 61$. Alternatively the sample size may be read from Table 13h in the row headed 15000 and column headed by 10.

The results of a particular choice of n and d^* can be shown graphically using what is called an operating characteristic (OC) curve where the variable on the horizontal axis is the proportion, P, in the population who have not been immunized. The vertical axis presents the probability of rejecting the null hypothesis H_0: $P=P_0$ and concluding that the vaccination coverage in the population is greater than P_0. Each combination of n and d^* will generate a unique curve. We know that if no one in the population is immunized then $P=1$ and there will be no chance of rejecting H_0. On the other hand, if everyone in the population is immunized then $P=0$ and we would always reject H_0. We look for rules which give us a very high probability of rejecting H_0 when there is a high coverage, i.e., P small. Fig. 10 presents a typical OC curve for $n=7$, $d^*=1$.

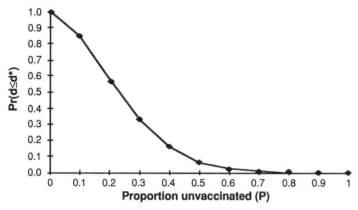

Fig. 10 Operating characteristic curve for $P_0=0.5$, $n=7$ and $d^*=1$

Additional curves can be constructed by varying n and d*. The power of the test is reflected in how steeply the curve rises to 1.0 in the region $0 \leq P \leq P_0$.

The choice of the final rule then comes down to one of combining the desired power, $1-\beta$, with the desired α level. Rather than providing curves which are difficult to read precisely, Tables 14a-14i, which present the values of (n,d*) pairs for chosen values of α, β, P_0 and P_a, have been developed.

In these tables, (n,d*) are chosen so that $\text{Prob}(d \leq d^* \mid n, P_0) \leq \alpha$ and $\text{Prob}(d \leq d^*+1 \mid n, P_0) > \alpha$. The LQAS survey problem is a one-sided test of $H_0: P = P_0$ versus $H_a: P = P_a$ where $P_a < P_0$, (i.e., it is a test of the hypothesis that the proportion nonimmunized is a specified level, versus the alternative that the proportion nonimmunized is less than the specified level). We first choose that sample size which will yield a test with stated α and β errors for the particular null and alternative hypothesis specified using formula (3) of Chapter 1. Use of this formula is based on the assumption that the normal approximation to the binomial is valid. The value of d* for the necessary n is determined by using the formula

$$d^* = [(nP_0) - z_{1-\alpha} \sqrt{\{nP_0(1-P_0)\}}], \tag{14}$$

$$\text{Prob}\{d \leq d^*\} = \sum_{d=0}^{d^*} \text{Prob}(d) = \sum_{d=0}^{d^*} [^nC_d] (P_0)^d (1-P_0)^{n-d}$$

where values of d* are always rounded down (e.g. [5.3] = 5; [6.8] = 6). When $n \leq 20$, d* is determined by exact computations with the binomial distribution.

Example I.5.1
A child-health program in a large refugee camp aims at reaching at least 70% of the children but it is feared that probably no more than 40% are being reached. How many children should be sampled to monitor the program's activities, and what should be the maximum acceptable number of children in the sample *not* reached by the program so as to test for the program's performance target, at the 5% level with a power of 80%?

Solution
The null hypothesis is: $P_0 = 0.70$ and the alternative is: $P_a = 0.40$ with a 5% level of significance and a power of 80% using formula (3), in Section 1, gives:

$$n = \{1.6449 \sqrt{[(0.70)(0.30)]} + 0.8416\sqrt{[(0.40)(0.60)]}\}^2/(0.30)^2$$
$$= 15.5$$

Therefore a random sample of 16 children would be needed. Using formula (14):

$$d^* = [(16)(0.70) - 1.6449 \sqrt{\{(16)(0.70)(0.30)\}}]$$
$$= 8.2$$

Out of the 16 children if 8 or more children are found *not* to have been reached by the program then the null hypothesis would be rejected and the conclusion would be that the program is behind its original target.

Alternatively, the values of n and d^* may be read from Table 14e in the row headed 40% and column headed 70%. Discrepancies between Table 14e and the results obtained with formula (14) are due to the more appropriate use of exact binomial calculations in Table 14e.

These tables clearly demonstrate the trade off one must make between power and sample size in LQAS surveys. It is essentially impossible to have $\alpha=0.05$, $\beta=0.2$ and use $n=5$ unless P_a under the alternative was actually close to 0. Hence investigators with limited resources must be ready to compromise on the value of β or the difference between P_0 and P_a. The more serious error of concluding that an inadequately immunized population has adequate coverage is being guarded against by the value of α which can always be controlled.

6 The incidence rate

In many epidemiologic studies it is useful to use a measure of disease occurrence which expresses the number of observed events relative to something other than the total number of persons at risk of the event. The most common of these alternative measures is the **incidence rate**. This measure has been called the **incidence density**, the **person-time incidence rate**, the **instantaneous incidence rate**, the **force of morbidity**, and the **hazard** by various authors. The measure expresses the number of events relative to the time over which they occur. It is an especially useful measure when one is interested in expressing the risk of disease relative to some unit of time.

The following example illustrates the calculation of the incidence rate, "λ", which is a population parameter and its estimate "$\hat{\lambda}$".

Suppose we have 5 individuals who are followed up for 5 years and 2 develop the event of interest, for example cardio-vascular disease (CVD), after 2 and 3 years of follow-up. Since the total number of events is 2 and the total person-years of risk is 5+5+5+2+3=20, the estimated incidence rate is

$$\hat{\lambda} = 2/20 = 0.1 \ .$$

This estimated rate is typically expressed in some multiple of persons per year. In this example the incidence rate can be expressed as 1 CVD case per 10 people per year. In other words, if we were to follow up 10 people for 1 year we would expect one of them to develop CVD.

The goals of a study using λ as the measure of interest might include estimating it to within a stated precision and/or testing whether it was equal to some specific value λ_0. These would be single-sample studies. Alternatively one may wish to test whether the incidence rates for two different populations are the same versus some specific alternative hypothesis.

Development of the sample size determination methods for the incidence rate studies is based on "survival analysis" based, in turn, on the hazard function. The methods of this field are extensive and include many different models. The reader is referred to the texts by Gross and Clark[26], Lee[39], Miller[51], and Kalbfleisch and Prentice[34] for a treatment of this field with health related applications. The hazard function gives the conditional probability that the event will occur in the next "instant" given that the event has not yet occurred. Expressing the hazard in different mathematical forms yields different survival distributions. For example, the probability that a 42 year old male will develop CVD in the next year given that he is free of the disease at his 42nd birthday is the hazard or incidence density for 42-year-old males. The notion of "an instant" may be as long as a year for some chronic diseases and as short as a day for some highly infectious diseases.

To develop the expressions needed for ascertainment of sample size, a model with the statistical distribution of survival times in the population following an exponential distribution, will be assumed. Under this model, the probability that an individual will survive for more than t time units is

$$S(t) = e^{-\lambda t}$$

and that the survival time is less than or equal to t is

$$P(t) = 1 - e^{-\lambda t} = 1 - S(t) .$$

The conditional probability that the individual will develop CVD in the forthcoming interval of unit length, given that the event has not yet occurred prior to that interval, is constant and equal to λ. In other words the hazard function for this model is constant and equal to λ. This assumption of constant success rate may not be appropriate for certain diseases or for large groups of individuals, but may be realistic for certain age-, sex- or race-specific groups. For example, the risk of CVD does not change dramatically for white males, in the USA., during the years 40-45. If μ denotes the mean survival time, then $\lambda = 1/\mu$.

If we consider the information on follow-up of the five individuals discussed in an earlier example, we note that two of these persons had developed CVD, by the end of the study. This type of observation, or in fact any observation of follow-up which is terminated before the event has occurred, is said to be **censored**. Under the assumption of exponential survival the maximum likelihood estimate of the hazard function is

$$\hat{\lambda} = d/F$$

(see Gross and Clark[26] Chapter 3) where d is the number of events and F is the total follow-up time. In the previous example, $d = 2$, $F = 20$ and $\hat{\lambda} = 0.1$. Thus, the incidence density is the estimate of the hazard under exponential survival. This result will provide the basis for development of formulae to determine necessary sample size. In many epidemiologic studies the hazard rate may change considerably with age although the assumption of a constant hazard may be approximately true during the time period considered in most studies.

Suppose we are planning an experiment which involves observing experimental subjects from the time they receive a "treatment" until a "success" occurs. (For example, the experimental subject may be a human, the treatment may be an analgesic, and success might be the end of a headache.) The subject is observed until "success" occurs; thus there is no censoring. Let $t_1,...,t_n$ represent the observed success times for the n subjects.

In this case $\hat{\lambda} = 1/t$, where

$$t = (1/n) \sum_{i=1}^{n} t_i.$$

It follows from the theory of maximum likelihood estimation that where n is sufficiently large, $\hat{\lambda}$ is normally distributed with mean λ and variance λ^2/n. This information may be used in the same way that similar information was used to develop sample size formulae for estimation and tests about proportions. The sample size which is necessary to estimate λ to within ε of its true value with probability $(1-\alpha)$ is given by the formula

$$n = [z_{1-\alpha/2}/\varepsilon]^2 \tag{15}$$

from $|\hat{\lambda}-\lambda| = z_{1-\alpha/2}[\lambda/\sqrt{n}]$ with $\varepsilon = |\hat{\lambda}-\lambda|/\lambda$. These values of n may be looked up directly in Table 15.

Example I.6.1
How many people should be followed-up to estimate the hazard (incidence rate) to within 10% of the true value with 95% confidence?

Solution

Using formula (15) with $\varepsilon = 0.10$ and $z = 1.960$ it follows that

$$n = (1.960/0.1)^2 = 384.16,$$

indicating that we would need to follow-up 385 individuals until the "success" time of each individual was known. This value may be found by using Table 15, at the intersection of the row corresponding to $\varepsilon=0.10$ and the column corresponding to the 95% confidence level.

In order to test a hypothesis about the hazard (incidence rate), we must consider formulation of the alternative hypothesis. The incidence rate expresses risk on the basis of events per so many persons per time unit. We may wish to state the null and alternative hypotheses directly. For example, H_0: $\lambda = 0.1$ versus H_a: $\lambda = 0.05$. Under H_a we have 5 events per 100 persons per time unit or 1/2 the incidence rate under H_0. Alternatively, the null and alternative hypothesis may be expressed in terms of the mean length of time to failure, μ, through the relationship $\mu = 1/\lambda$. For example, when $\lambda = 0.1$, $\mu = 1/0.1 = 10$. In the alternative we might express our belief that the mean length of time to failure will be 15 (this would correspond to $\lambda = 1/15 = 0.06667$). Since the expression of the null and alternative hypothesis in terms of μ or λ is equally satisfactory, the decision should be based on whichever is most biologically meaningful for the problem at hand. This will depend on the available data. If incidence data are available, λ_0 and λ_a should be specified directly; otherwise λ_0 and λ_a should be specified indirectly through μ_0 and μ_a. The test statistic for H_0: $\lambda=\lambda_0$ is

$$z = (\hat{\lambda}-\lambda_0)(\sqrt{n})/\lambda_0$$

which is distributed $N(0,1)$ under the null hypothesis. To obtain an expression for the necessary sample size which will detect the two-sided alternative H_a: $\lambda \neq \lambda_0$ with stated power, we must find that value of n such that

$$\text{Prob}\{(\hat{\lambda}-\lambda_0)\sqrt{n}/\lambda_0 > z_{1-\alpha/2} | H_a\} = 1-\beta.$$

Using a strategy similar to the one used in developing the formula for the sample size for hypothesis testing for a single population proportion, Fig. 3 and equation (4), gives:

$$\lambda_0 + z_{1-\alpha/2} [\lambda_0/\sqrt{n}] = \lambda_a - z_{1-\beta} [\lambda_a/\sqrt{n}].$$

Solving for n, it follows that

$$n = \frac{(z_{1-\alpha/2}\lambda_0 + z_{1-\beta}\lambda_a)^2}{(\lambda_0-\lambda_a)^2} \qquad (16)$$

Tables 16a-16i provide sample sizes based on formula (16). The appropriate sample size is located in the table, for specified α and β levels, at the intersection of the row representing λ_a and the column representing λ_0.

Example I.6.2

Suppose it is widely reported that the hazard due to a certain chemical exposure in a particular industry had always been 0.20, but, recently with the introduction of new production techniques the hazard has been changed by 25%. How many people should be followed-up to test H_0: $\lambda_0 = 0.20$ versus $\lambda_a = 0.15$ or 0.25 at the 5% level of significance and with 80% power?

Solution

Using formula (16) with $\lambda_0 = 0.20$; $\lambda_a = 0.15$ or 0.25; $z_{1-\alpha/2} = 1.960$ and $z_{1-\beta} = 0.842$ it follows that

$$n = (1.960 \times 0.20 + 0.842 \times 0.15)^2/(0.05)^2$$
$$= 107.45$$

or

$$n = (1.960 \times 0.20 + 0.842 \times 0.25)^2/(0.05)^2$$
$$= 145.20$$

Therefore 146 people would have to be followed-up. These results could have been obtained from Table 16e by taking the larger of the two numbers given in the column headed 0.20 and rows headed 0.15 and 0.25.

In the above example, under the null hypothesis the average time to follow-up is $\mu_0 = 1/\lambda_0 = 5$ "years" and under the alternative it is $\mu_a = 1/\lambda_a = 4$ or 6.7 "years" depending on whether $\lambda_a > \lambda_0$ or $\lambda_a < \lambda_0$. Thus the study could take up to nearly 7 "years" to complete if the unit of time for the study is in years. This points out the problem of not allowing for censoring. We need few subjects but it requires a long time to complete. Modifications in the study design based on control of the follow-up period will now be presented for the two-sample problem.

Typically, an investigator will be interested in comparing the incidence rate in two populations. In this situation the goal is usually to test the null hypothesis $H_0: \lambda_1 = \lambda_2$ (or, $H_0: \lambda_1 - \lambda_2 = 0$) rather than to estimate the difference with stated precision. Hence sample size formulae will be developed only for the hypothesis testing situation.

Consider the situation in which each subject is followed until the event of interest is observed. The null hypothesis is stated as $H_0: \lambda_1 - \lambda_2 = 0$ and the two-sided alternative is $H_a: \lambda_1 - \lambda_2 \neq 0$, where both λ_1 and λ_2 are specified under H_a. The methodology for selecting the values of λ_1 and λ_2 is identical to that used in the single-sample case. The test statistic is

$$z = \frac{(\hat{\lambda}_1 - \hat{\lambda}_2)}{\sqrt{2\bar{\lambda}^2/2}} = \frac{(\hat{\lambda}_1 - \hat{\lambda}_2)\sqrt{n}}{\bar{\lambda}\sqrt{2}}$$

where $\bar{\lambda} = (\hat{\lambda}_1 + \hat{\lambda}_2)/2$ assuming equal group sizes. We must find that value of n such that

$$\text{Prob}\{ z > z_{1-\alpha/2} | H_a \} = 1-\beta .$$

Using the same method as was used in developing formula (7) for the sample size for hypothesis testing for two population proportions, and Fig. 4 (replacing $P_1 - P_2$ with $\lambda_1 - \lambda_2$) gives:

$$z_{1-\alpha/2}\sqrt{[2\bar{\lambda}^2/n]} = (\lambda_1 - \lambda_2) - z_{1-\beta}\sqrt{[(\lambda_1^2 + \lambda_2^2)/n]} .$$

Then, solving for n it follows that

$$n = \frac{\{z_{1-\alpha/2}\sqrt{[2\bar{\lambda}^2]} + z_{1-\beta}\sqrt{[\lambda_1^2 + \lambda_2^2]}\}^2}{(\lambda_1 - \lambda_2)^2} \qquad (17)$$

Tables 17a-17i provide sample sizes based on formula (17). The appropriate sample size is located in the table, for specified α and β levels, at the intersection of the row representing λ_2 and the column representing λ_1.

If there are to be unequal sample sizes, n_1 and n_2, from the two populations, then formula (17) generalizes to:

$$n_1 = \frac{\{z_{1-\alpha/2}\sqrt{[(1+k)\bar{\lambda}^2]} + z_{1-\beta}\sqrt{[k\lambda_1{}^2+\lambda_2{}^2]}\}^2}{k(\lambda_1-\lambda_2)^2} \qquad (17a)$$

with $\bar{\lambda}=(\hat{\lambda}_1 + k\hat{\lambda}_2)/(1+k)$ where $k = n_2/n_1$. Tables 17a-17i cover the most common situation of $k=1$.

Example I.6.3
Suppose that a disease hazard due to a certain chemical exposure in a particular industry is believed to be roughly 0.10 and a competing industry uses techniques with a disease hazard believed to be roughly 0.05, how many people would be needed to be followed-up in each industrial exposure to test, at the 5% level of significance with a power of 80%, whether there is a difference in the disease hazards in the two industries?

Solution
Using formula (17) with $\bar{\lambda} = (0.1+ 0.05)/2 = 0.075$ yields

$$n = \frac{\left\{1.960\sqrt{2(0.075)^2} +0.842\sqrt{(0.1)^2+(0.05)^2}\right\}^2}{(0.1 -0.05)^2} =36.49$$

Hence, at least 37 subjects would have to be followed-up in each group until the event/failure occurs. This value may be found as the first entry in Table 17e.

An alternative strategy is to begin the study on a fixed date, allow patients to enroll in the study throughout the period, and terminate enrollment and follow up for "T" years. This controls the time duration of the study but we must worry about how to account for the censored observations which are bound to occur. The mathematical details of the necessary modifications to formula (17) are sketched in the papers by Donner[12] and Lachin[37] and developed more fully in Gross and Clark[26]. The modification of formula (17) requires that we evaluate

$$f(\lambda) = \lambda^3 T/(\lambda T - 1 + e^{-\lambda T})$$

and use the following formula for n:

$$n = \frac{\{z_{1-\alpha/2}\sqrt{[2f(\bar{\lambda})]} + z_{1-\beta}\sqrt{[f(\lambda_1)+f(\lambda_2)]}\}^2}{(\lambda_1-\lambda_2)^2} \qquad (18)$$

Example I.6.4
Consider the data in Example I.6.3 with the additional limitation that the study will terminate in 5 years. We wish to test H_0: $\lambda_1 = \lambda_2 = 0.1$ versus the alternative that H_a: $\lambda_1 = 0.1$, $\lambda_2 = 0.05$ with $\alpha = 0.05$, $\beta = 0.2$. How many people should be followed up?

Solution
Using the formula for $f(\lambda)$:

$$f(\bar{\lambda} = 0.075) = 0.0339$$

$f(\lambda_1 = 0.1)$ $= 0.0469$
$f(\lambda_2 = 0.05)$ $= 0.0217$

and

$n = \{1.960 \sqrt{[2(0.0339)]} + 0.8416 \sqrt{[0.0469 + 0.0217]}\}^2/(0.1-0.05)^2$
$= 213.7$

By restricting the study duration to 5 years we need many more subjects (214) in each group than was previously the case. The reason for this is that the average time to failure is 10 years under H_0 and 20 years under H_a, . The survival rates are too high to be realistic for a 5 year study.

Example I.6.5
Suppose that the average survival for patients suffering from a specific disease and receiving a standard treatment is 2 years but there is a new treatment which will receive approval for marketing if it can be demonstrated that it would increase the patients' survival, on average, by at least 1 year; how many subjects would a 5 -year study require?

Solution
In this example $\lambda_1 = 0.5$, $\lambda_2 = 0.33$ and $\bar{\lambda} = 0.4167$

$f(\bar{\lambda} = 0.4167)$ $= 0.2995$
$f(\lambda_1 = 0.5)$ $= 0.3950$
$f(\lambda_2 = 0.33)$ $= 0.2164$

and

$n = \{1.645\sqrt{[2(0.2995)]} + 0.842\sqrt{[0.3950 + 0.2164]}\}^2/(0.5 - 0.33)^2$
$=163.74$

Thus 164 subjects would be needed in each group. If, however, the follow-up was uncensored 100 subjects would be needed in each group.

Examples I.6.4 and I.6.5 illustrate that the proposed length of the study cannot be chosen with total disregard to the survival times that are likely to be observed.

Using the results presented in Gross and Clark[26], Lachin[37] has extended formula (18) to cover the situation in which subjects are enrolled for T_1 years and the total duration of the study is T years. .

The following formula is used for n:

$$n = \frac{\{z_{1-\alpha/2}\sqrt{[2g(\bar{\lambda})]} + z_{1-\beta}\sqrt{[g(\lambda_1)+g(\lambda_2)]}\}^2}{(\lambda_1-\lambda_2)^2} \qquad (19)$$

where

$$g(\lambda) = \lambda^3 T_1/[\lambda T_1 - e^{-\lambda(T-T_1)} + e^{-\lambda T}]$$

Example I.6.6
Suppose, in Example I.6.5, that subjects are to be enrolled in the study for 2.5 years and then continue the follow-up for another 2.5 years, how many people would have to be included in the study?

Solution
With $T_1 = 2.5$, $T = 5$, $\lambda_1 = 0.5$, $\lambda_2 = 0.3333$ and $\bar{\lambda} = 0.4167$ yields

$g(\bar{\lambda} = 0.4167)$ $= 0.2224$

$$g\,(\lambda_1 = 0.5000) \;\; = 0.2989$$
$$g\,(\lambda_2 = 0.3333) \;\; = 0.1576$$

Then using formula (19)

$$n = \{1.645\sqrt{[2(0.2224)]} \;+\; 0.842\;\sqrt{[0.2989 \;+\; 0.1576]}\}^2/(0.5-0.3333)^2$$
$$= 99.88$$

Thus only 100 subjects would be needed in each group if the design allowed for 2.5 years of follow-up after an enrollment period of 2.5 years. The saving of subjects occurs because all subjects are being followed for at least 2.5 years, which is the average survival time under H_0 and H_a. Thus we expect to observe many more failures/events. The precision of the study depends on the expected number of events. The design which generates the greatest number of events over the shortest enrollment and follow-up period will require the fewest overall number of participants.

The development of formulae for sample size involving incidence rates was framed entirely in the domain of survival studies. Examples of these in health research include most clinical trials of cancer therapies. The results are easily interpreted in this context. The extension to other types of studies comes from the observation that the measure, incidence density, or person-years incidence, is an estimate of a hazard function under exponential survival. This assumption will be approximately valid for relatively homogeneous groups of subjects.

Finally, the use of the incidence density ratio (IDR) as a measure of comparing two populations will, under certain conditions, be as an approximation to the relative risk. In the notation of this Chapter, the test of the hypothesis that $\lambda_1 = \lambda_2$ is fully equivalent to a test that the IDR $= \lambda_1/\lambda_2 = 1$. Direct tests about the ratio would be based on $\ln(\text{IDR}) = \ln(\lambda_1)-\ln(\lambda_2)$. Sample sizes based on the distribution theory of $\ln(\lambda_1)-\ln(\lambda_2)$ will not differ significantly from the sample sizes obtained from equations (17), (18), and (19), which are likely to be accurate enough for most purposes.

7 Sample size for continuous response variables

Many of the sample size issues developed so far for binary random variables and the associated methods for inference concerning the population proportion can be extended for application to continuous random variables and parameters such as population means and totals. In this Chapter we present some of the formulae necessary to determine sample sizes for estimating and testing hypotheses about the population mean.

The one-sample problem

Estimating the population mean

We denote the true but unknown mean in the population by "μ" and unknown variance by σ^2. By the central limit theorem, the sampling distribution of the sample mean "$\bar{x}$" is approximately normal with mean $E(\bar{x})=\mu$, and variance $Var(\bar{x})=\sigma^2/n$. We define the quantity d as the distance, in either direction, from the true population mean,

$$d = z_{1-\alpha/2}\sqrt{(\sigma^2/n)} \, ,$$

where $z_{1-\alpha/2}$ represents the number of standard errors from the mean. As before, d is the **precision** of the estimate and can be made as small as desired by increasing the sample size n. Specifically, if $z_{1-\alpha/2}$ is chosen to be 1.960, then 95% of all sample means will fall within 1.960 standard errors of the population mean μ, where a standard error equals $\sqrt{(\sigma^2/n)}$. Solving the above expression for n it follows that

$$n = \frac{z_{1-\alpha/2}^2 \sigma^2}{d^2} \tag{20}$$

This expression depends upon the unknown population parameter σ^2 which could be estimated from a pilot sample or other available sources.

Example I.7.1
Suppose an estimate is desired of the average retail price of twenty tablets of a commonly used tranquilizer. A random sample of retail pharmacies is to be selected. The estimate is required to be within 10 cents of the true average price with 95% confidence. Based on a small pilot study, the standard deviation in price, σ, can be estimated as 85 cents. How many pharmacies should be randomly selected?

Solution
Using the above formula, it follows that

$$n = [(1.960)^2(0.85)^2]/(0.10)^2 = 277.56.$$

As a result, a sample of 278 pharmacies should be taken.

In this example, it might seem more reasonable to require that the estimate of μ fall within 10% of μ rather than to within a specified number of units of μ. The formula used for this purpose is:

$$n = \frac{z_{1-\alpha/2}^2 \sigma^2}{\varepsilon^2 \mu^2} \tag{21}$$

Example I.7.2
Consider the data in Example I.7.1, but this time we will determine the sample size necessary to be 95% confident of estimating the average retail price of twenty tablets of the tranquilizer in the population of all pharmacies to within 5% (not 10 cents) of the true value, if, based on the pilot survey data, we believe that the true price should be about $1.00.

Solution
Assuming $\sigma^2=(0.85)^2$, and using formula (21) above,

$$n = [(1.960)^2(0.85)^2]/[(0.05)^2(1.00)^2] = 1110.22.$$

Hence 1111 pharmacies should be sampled in order to be 95% confident that the resulting estimate will fall between $0.95 and $1.05 if the true average price is $1.00.

In the above situations, our primary aim was estimation of the population mean. We now consider sample size determination when there is an underlying hypothesis which is to be tested.

Hypothesis testing - one population mean

Suppose we would like to test the hypothesis

$$H_0: \mu = \mu_0$$

versus the alternative hypothesis

$$H_a: \mu > \mu_0$$

and we would like to fix the level of the type I error to equal α and the type II error to equal β. That is, we want the power of the test to equal $1-\beta$. Without loss of generality, we will denote the actual μ in the population as μ_a. Following the same development as was done with respect to hypothesis testing for the population proportion (with the additional assumption that the variance of $\bar{x}$ is equal to σ^2/n under both H_0 and H_a), the necessary sample size for this single-sample hypothesis testing situation is given by the formula:

$$n = \frac{\sigma^2[z_{1-\alpha} + z_{1-\beta}]^2}{[\mu_0 - \mu_a]^2} \tag{22}$$

Example I.7.3
A survey had indicated that the average weight of men over 55 years of age with newly diagnosed heart disease was 90 kg. However, it is suspected that the average weight of such men is now somewhat lower. How large a sample would be necessary to test, at the 5% level of significance with a power of 90%, whether the average weight is unchanged versus the alternative that it has decreased from 90 to 85 kg with an estimated standard deviation of 20 kg?

Solution
Using formula (22):

$$n = 20^2(1.645+1.282)^2/(90-85)^2 = 137.08.$$

Therefore, a sample of 138 men over 55 years of age with newly diagnosed heart disease would be required.

Note that, as was the case for population proportions, in order to calculate n, α, β, μ_0 and

μ_a must be specified. A similar approach is followed when the alternative is two-sided. That is, when we wish to test

$$H_0: \mu = \mu_0$$

versus

$$H_a: \mu \neq \mu_0.$$

In this situation, the null hypothesis is rejected if $\bar{x}$ is too large or too small. We assign area $\alpha/2$ to each tail of the sampling distribution under H_0. The only adjustment to formula (22) is that $z_{1-\alpha/2}$ is used in place of $z_{1-\alpha}$ resulting in

$$n = \frac{\sigma^2 [z_{1-\alpha/2} + z_{1-\beta}]^2}{[\mu_0-\mu_a]^2} \tag{23}$$

Example I.7.4
A two-sided test of Example I.7.3 could be designed to test the hypothesis that the average weight has not changed versus the alternative that the average weight has changed, and that a difference of 5 kg would be considered important.

Solution
Using formula (23) with $z_{1-\alpha/2} = 1.960$, $z_{1-\beta} = 1.282$ and $\sigma = 20$,

$$n = 20^2(1.960+1.282)^2/(5)^2 = 168.17.$$

Thus, 169 men would be required for the sample if the alternative were two-sided.

The two-sample problem

We now focus on estimating the difference between two population means and on testing hypotheses concerning the equality of means in two groups.

Estimating the difference between two means
The difference between two population means represents a new parameter, $\mu_1-\mu_2$. An estimate of this parameter is given by the difference in the sample means, $\bar{x}_1-\bar{x}_2$. The mean of the sampling distribution of $\bar{x}_1-\bar{x}_2$ is

$$E(\bar{x}_1-\bar{x}_2) = \mu_1-\mu_2$$

and the variance of this distribution is

$$Var(\bar{x}_1-\bar{x}_2) = Var(\bar{x}_1) + Var(\bar{x}_2) = \sigma_1^2/n_1 + \sigma_2^2/n_2 .$$

For simplicity, we will assume that $\sigma_1^2=\sigma_2^2=\sigma^2$. Under this assumption we say the variances are said to be **homoskedastic** and the formula for the variance of the difference can be simplified to

$$Var(\bar{x}_1-\bar{x}_2) = \sigma^2/n_1 + \sigma^2/n_2 = \sigma^2 (1/n_1 + 1/n_2) .$$

The value σ^2 is an unknown population parameter, which can be estimated from sample or pilot data by pooling the individual sample variances, s_1^2 and s_2^2, to form the **pooled variance**, s_p^2, where

$$s_p^2 = \frac{(n_1-1)\, s_1^2 + (n_2-1)\, s_2^2}{(n_1-1)+(n_2-1)}$$

where n_1 and n_2 are the sample sizes in the pilot study.

If, in addition, the same number of observations is selected from each of the two populations ($n_1=n_2=n$), then

$$\text{Var}(\bar{x}_1 - \bar{x}_2) = \sigma^2/n + \sigma^2/n = 2\sigma^2/n .$$

Following the same logic used in estimating a single population mean, the quantity d denotes the distance, in either direction, from the population difference, $\mu_1-\mu_2$, and may be expressed as

$$d = z_{1-\alpha/2} \sqrt{[2\sigma^2/n]} .$$

Solving this expression for n it follows that

$$n = \frac{z_{1-\alpha/2}^2 [2\sigma^2]}{d^2} \qquad\qquad (24)$$

Example I.7.5
Nutritionists wish to estimate the difference in caloric intake at lunch between children in a school offering a hot school lunch program and children in a school which does not. From other nutrition studies, they estimate that the standard deviation in caloric intake among elementary school children is 75 calories, and they wish to make their estimate to within 20 calories of the true difference with 95% confidence.

Solution
Using formula (24) ,

$$n=(1.960)^2[2(75^2)]/20^2=108.05.$$

Thus, 109 children from each school should be studied.

Hypothesis testing for two population means
Suppose a study is designed to test $H_0: \mu_1=\mu_2$ versus $H_a: \mu_1>\mu_2$. The mean of the sampling distribution of $\bar{x}_1 - \bar{x}_2$ under H_0 is 0 and the variance is

$$\text{Var}(\bar{x}_1 - \bar{x}_2) = 2\sigma^2/n .$$

Now, suppose we would like to know how many observations to take in order to be $100(1-\alpha)\%$ confident of rejecting H_0 when, in fact, the true difference between the population means is $(\mu_1-\mu_2) = \delta$.

Following a strategy similar to that employed in developing formula (7), it follows that

$$n = \frac{2\sigma^2[z_{1-\alpha/2}+z_{1-\beta}]^2}{(\mu_1-\mu_2)^2} \qquad\qquad (25)$$

Since the value of σ^2 would not ordinarily be known, it could be estimated from a pilot study using s_p^2. The quantity $\mu_1-\mu_2$ represents that difference considered to be of sufficient practical significance to warrant detection.

Example I.7.6

Suppose a study is being designed to measure the effect, on systolic blood pressure, of lowering sodium in the diet. From a pilot study it is observed that the standard deviation of systolic blood pressure in a community with a high sodium diet is 12 mmHg while that in a group with a low sodium diet is 10.3 mmHg. If $\alpha=0.05$ and $\beta=0.10$, how large a sample from each community should be selected if we want to be able to detect a 2 mmHg difference in blood pressure between the two communities?

Solution

Pooling the two variances, $s_p^2 = [s_1^2+s_2^2]/2 = [144.0+106.1]/2 = 125.05$. (This computation assumes that the pilot study used equal sample sizes, otherwise a weighted average would be used.) This value is used in place of σ^2 in formula (25) to test

$$H_0: \mu_1-\mu_2=0$$

versus

$$H_a: \mu_1-\mu_2\neq0$$

where, specifically, $\mu_1-\mu_2 = 2$ is used as the alternative. This gives:

$$n = 2(125.05)[1.960+1.282]^2/2^2 = 657.17.$$

Hence, a sample of 658 subjects would be needed in each of the two groups.

A similar approach is followed when the alternative is one-sided. That is, testing $H_0:\mu_1-\mu_2=0$ versus $H_a:\mu_1-\mu_2>0$. The sample size necessary in this situation is

$$n = \frac{2\sigma^2[z_{1-\alpha}+z_{1-\beta}]^2}{(\mu_1-\mu_2)^2} \tag{26}$$

Example I.7.7

A study is being planned to test whether a dietary supplement for pregnant women will increase the birthweight of babies. One group of women will receive the new supplement and the other group will receive the usual nutrition consultation. From a pilot study, the standard deviation in birthweight is estimated at 500 g and is assumed to be the same for both groups. The hypothesis of no difference is to be tested at the 5% level of significance. It is desired to have 80% power ($\beta=0.20$) of detecting an increase of 100 g.

Solution

Using formula (26) it follows that

$$n = 2(500)^2[1.645+0.842]^2/(100)^2 = 309.26.$$

Hence, a sample of 310 subjects should be studied in each of the two groups.

Because of the wide range of possible parameter values, it is not possible to present a comprehensive set of sample size tables. Rather than provide a limited number of tables, only the formulae are presented.

8 Sample size for sample surveys

In designing sample surveys, one of the most important considerations is to assure that estimates obtained will be reliable[p] enough to meet the objectives of the survey. Specification of the desired level of reliability for resulting estimates is, therefore, an important first step in the planning process. In general, irrespective of the type of design employed, the larger the sample, the greater will be the reliability of the resulting estimate. Validity, on the other hand, is a function of the measurement process and will not be affected by sample size. Instead, validity can be improved by improving the techniques of data collection and management.

A sample survey generally has as its primary objective the estimation of an unknown population parameter θ with a given precision. A sample survey, irrespective of whether it is a simple random, stratified or cluster sample, and irrespective of whether the sampling takes place in one or multiple stages, produces an estimate $\hat{\theta}$ of θ along with an estimate of the variance of $\hat{\theta}$, denoted by $\text{Var}(\hat{\theta})$. There are two ways of expressing the desired precision of the estimate. The first specifies that $\hat{\theta}$ should not differ from θ by more than "d" units with $100(1-\alpha)\%$ confidence. The second specifies that we wish to be $100(1-\alpha)\%$ confident that our estimate $\hat{\theta}$ will not differ, in absolute value, from the true unknown population parameter, θ, by more than $\varepsilon\theta$. That is,

$$|\hat{\theta}-\theta|/\theta < \varepsilon .$$

Consider the case where θ is a population proportion, P. By applying the central limit theorem, and provided that the sample size is reasonably large, the sampling distribution of $\hat{P}$ may be approximated by the normal distribution. This can be illustrated in the following diagram:

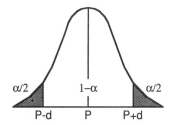

Fig. 11 Sampling distribution of $\hat{P}$

To determine the required sample size, d is set equal to the desired precision. That is, d may either be specified in terms of the number of percentage points or it may be specified as a percentage of P, i.e., $d=\varepsilon P$.

Irrespective of which sampling scheme is used, $\text{V}\hat{\text{a}}\text{r}(\hat{P})$ depends upon n, and determination of sample size simply involves setting up the formula

$$d = z_{1-\alpha/2}\sqrt{\text{V}\hat{\text{a}}\text{r}(\hat{P})} ,$$

substituting in the appropriate expression for $\text{V}\hat{\text{a}}\text{r}(\hat{P})$, and solving for n.

---

[p] See pages 61-63

Simple random and systematic sampling

With simple random or systematic sampling, the population proportion P is estimated by $\hat{P}^q$, where

$$\hat{P} = \sum_1^n y_i/n,$$

where $y_i = 0$ if the ith sampling unit does not have the characteristic,
or, $y_i = 1$ if the ith sampling unit does have the characteristicand the variance of $\hat{P}$ is given by

$$Var(\hat{P}) = \frac{P(1-P)}{n} \times \frac{N-n}{N-1}.$$

It should be noted that this expression incorporates the **finite population correction** ({N-n}/{N-1}), since, in most sample surveys, N is known and reflects the number of potential sampling units. In practice, since n is usually small relative to N, the correction is close to 1. If the finite population correction is not used in the formula, the calculated variance will be too large, yielding wider than necessary confidence intervals and/or larger than necessary sample sizes.

Estimating P to within "d" percentage points

Following the above stated strategy,

$$d = z_{1-\alpha/2}\sqrt{\{[P(1-P)(N-n)]/[n(N-1)]\}}$$

and solving for n it follows that

$$n = \frac{z^2_{1-\alpha/2}P(1-P) \cdot N}{d^2(N-1) + z^2_{1-\alpha/2}P(1-P)}. \qquad (27)$$

This formula may be simplified somewhat if we assume that the sample size n will be small relative to a rather large population size N. Then the expression (N-n)/(N-1) in the formula for $Var(\hat{P})$ may be considered equal to 1, the expression simplifies to

$$Var(\hat{P}) = P(1-P)/n,$$

and the sample size may be taken to equal

$$n = \frac{z^2_{1-\alpha/2}P(1-P)}{d^2} \qquad (28)$$

This expression is the same as formula (1) and, therefore, Tables 1a-1c present these sample sizes. If the population size N is known (which it will be with simple random sampling), the formula provides the correct sample size which often will not differ appreciably from formula (1). Hence, Table 1 may often be used as a quick

---

q See pages 53-54

approximation for formula (27). No tables are presented corresponding to formula (27) since the potential range of N is so great that it would not be possible to construct a concise table.

Example I.8.1
A preliminary random sample of 50 children is selected from 4000 children living in a particular village and it is found that 30 of them have ascariasis. How large a sample must be selected to be 95% confident that the estimate of P will not differ from the true P by more that 5 percentage points?

Solution
Using the 50 children as a pilot sample in order to estimate P for use in formula (27) it follows that

$$n = [4000(1.960)^2(0.6)(0.4)]/[(0.05)^2(3999)+(1.960)^2(0.6)(0.4)] = 337.74.$$

Hence a simple random sample of 338 children should be selected, which means that an additional 288 children should be studied. Alternatively, using the simpler formula (1), it follows that

$$n = (1.960)^2(0.6)(0.4)/(0.05)^2 = 368.79,$$

suggesting that a total sample of 369 children should be studied. This value may also be found in Table 1b at the intersection of the column headed 0.40, and the row headed 5%.

Estimating P to within "ε" of P

Following the alternate strategy, we set

$$\varepsilon P = z_{1-\alpha/2} \sqrt{\{[P(1-P)(N-n)]/[n(N-1)]\}}$$

and solving for n it follows that

$$n = \frac{z_{1-\alpha/2}^2 N(1-P)}{\varepsilon^2 P(n-1) + z_{1-\alpha/2}^2(1-P)} \tag{29}$$

If we assume that N is large and much greater than n, then the simplified expression for the estimated variance results in the following expression for n

$$n = \frac{z_{1-\alpha/2}^2(1-P)}{\varepsilon^2 P} \tag{29a}$$

which may be recognized as formula (2) of this manual. The sample sizes based on this simplified expression are given in Tables 2a-2c.

Example I.8.2
Suppose, in Example I.8.1, we wish to estimate the proportion of children in the population with ascariasis to within 5% of the true value with 95% confidence, how many children should be sampled?

Solution
Using formula (29), it follows that

$$n = [1.960^2(4000)(1-0.6)]/[0.05^2(0.6)(3999)+1.960^2(1-0.6)] = 815.72.$$

Hence an additional 766 children would be studied to obtain a total sample of 816 children. Alternatively, using the simplified formula (29a),

$$n = 1.960^2(1-0.6)/[(0.05)^2(0.6)] = 1024.43.$$

This required sample size of 1025 children may also be found in Table 2b at the intersection of the row headed 5% and the column headed 0.60.

Stratified random sampling[r]

In stratified random sampling, the population is divided into "L" strata, and simple random samples are selected from each such stratum. The proportion of individuals in the population who possess the characteristic of interest is

$$P = \sum_{h=1}^{L} N_h P_h/N ,$$

where P_h is the proportion of individuals in stratum h possessing the characteristic. That is, the population proportion is a weighted average of the stratum-specific proportions, where the weights are the relative sizes of strata, N_h.

An unbiased estimate of P is obtained by computing

$$\hat{P} = \sum_{h=1}^{L} N_h \hat{P}_h/N ,$$

where $\hat{P}_h$ is the usual estimate of P_h based on the n_h sampling units selected from the hth stratum.

The variance of the estimated proportion is

$$Var(\hat{P}) = (1/N^2)\sum_{h=1}^{L} N_h^2[(N_h-n_h)/(N_h-1)][P_h(1-P_h)/n_h].$$

Finally, if we assume that the N_h are large and much greater than n_h, then this expression simplifies to

$$Var(\hat{P}) = (1/N^2)\sum_{h=1}^{L} N_h^2[P_h(1-P_h)/n_h].$$

Again, by applying the central limit theorem, the sampling distribution of $\hat{P}$ may be approximated by the normal distribution and, as a result, the precision may be set to d which again may be specified either in terms of a defined distance or as a percentage of P.

Estimating P to within "d" percentage points
Under the simplifying assumptions presented above, the sample size n required to estimate P to within d percentage points with $100(1-\alpha)\%$ confidence is

---

[r] See pages 82-83

$$n = \frac{z_{1-\alpha/2}^2 \sum_{h=1}^{L} [N_h^2 P_h(1-P_h)/w_h]}{N^2 d^2 + z_{1-\alpha/2}^2 \sum_{h=1}^{L} N_h P_h(1-P_h)} \qquad (30)$$

where $w_h = n_h/n$. That is, w_h is the fraction of observations allocated to stratum h and is typically decided in advance of sampling by the particular allocation scheme used. Thus, if **equal allocation** is used, then $w_h = 1/L$ for all strata. Alternatively, if **proportional allocation** is used, then $w_h = N_h/N$ for the hth stratum. Other types of allocation strategies are commonly employed (for instance, the ones that incorporate such features as variability in the strata and differential costs of sampling within the strata) but will not be discussed further in this manual.

Using the simplified formula for Var($\hat{P}$) results in a somewhat simpler formula for sample size determination:

$$n = \frac{z_{1-\alpha/2}^2 \sum_{h=1}^{L} [N_h^2 P_h(1-P_h)/w_h]}{N^2 d^2} \qquad (30a)$$

The number of combinations of parameters in these equations makes the construction of tables impractical. The interested reader would be well advised to use a programmable calculator or a spreadsheet program on a microcomputer to assist with the calculations.

Example I.8.3
A preliminary survey is made of 3 cities, A, B, and C with population sizes 2000, 3000, and 5000, respectively. The proportion of families with 1 or more infant deaths within the last 5 years is estimated and presented in Table I.2 as p_h. Using these preliminary data, determine the sample size which would be needed to estimate the proportion of families with infant deaths if the precision is to be within ±3 percentage points of the true population P with 95% confidence and the sample is to be distributed using proportional allocation.

Table I.2 Sample size computation by spreadsheet technique

City	\multicolumn{3}{c}{Population weight}			\multicolumn{4}{c}{Proportion}	
	N_h	w_h	N_h^2	p_h	$N_h p_h$	$N_h p_h(1-p_h)$	$N_h^2 p_h(1-p_h)/w_h$
A	2000	0.2	4000000	0.10	200	180.0	1800000
B	3000	0.3	9000000	0.15	450	382.5	3825000
C	5000	0.5	25000000	0.20	1000	800.0	8000000
Total	10000					1362.5	13625000

Solution
Using formula (30) it follows that

$$n = 1.960^2[13625000]/\{(10000)^2(0.03)^2 + 1.960^2(1362.5)\} = 549.61$$

Hence, a total sample of 550 families should be selected. With proportional allocation, the sample would be distributed to the three strata as follows:

$$n_1 = 550 \times 2000/10000 = 110,$$

$$n_2 = 550 \times 3000/10000 = 165,$$
$$n_3 = 550 \times 5000/10000 = 275.$$

Using formula (30a) results in

$$n = 1.960^2[13625000]/\{(10000)^2(0.03)^2\} = 581.58$$

which suggests that a sample of size 582 be used. Hence by using formula (30) which incorporates the finite population correction factors within each stratum, a reduced estimate of sample size is obtained.

Estimating P to within "ε" of P

For the alternative strategy, we set

$$\varepsilon P = z_{1-\alpha/2}\sqrt{\mathrm{Var}(\hat{P})}$$

and solving for n, noting that $NP = \Sigma N_h P_h$, it follows that

$$n = \frac{z_{1-\alpha/2}^2 \displaystyle\sum_{h=1}^{L} [N_h^2 P_h(1-P_h)/w_h}{\varepsilon^2 \left(\displaystyle\sum_{h=1}^{L} N_h P_h\right)^2 + z_{1-\alpha/2}^2 \displaystyle\sum_{h=1}^{L} N_h P_h(1-P_h)} \tag{31}$$

If we assume that N_h is large and much greater than n_h, then the simplified expression for Var(P) may be used, giving rise to the following, less complicated, sample size formula:

$$n = \frac{z_{1-\alpha/2}^2 \displaystyle\sum_{h=1}^{L} [N_h^2 P_h(1-P_h)/w_h}{\varepsilon^2 \left(\displaystyle\sum_{h=1}^{L} N_h P_h\right)^2} \tag{31a}$$

Example I.8.4
In Example I.8.3, suppose that we wish to estimate P to within 5% of the true value how large a sample should be used?

Solution
Using the calculations in Table I.2 and formula (31):

$$n = 1.960^2[13625000]/\{(0.05)^2(1650)^2 + 1.960^2(1362.5)\} = 4347.17.$$

Hence, a sample of 4348 families should be selected. Since we are using proportional allocation, the sample would be distributed to the three strata as follows:

$$n_1 = 4348 \times 2000/10000 = 870,$$
$$n_2 = 4348 \times 3000/10000 = 1304,$$
$$n_3 = 4348 \times 5000/10000 = 2174.$$

Using formula (31a) results in:

$$n = 1.960^2[13625000]/\{(0.05)^2(1650)^2\} = 7690.26$$

which suggests that a sample of size 7691 be used. Hence by using formula (31) which incorporates the finite population correction factors within each stratum, a greatly reduced estimate of the sample size requirement was obtained.

There is no easy rule to give for deciding upon sample size for cluster sampling. The easiest approach is to compute n based on simple random sampling criteria and then multiply by the design effect[s] to obtain the required *total* sample with cluster sampling. If 2 were the chosen design effect, twice as many observations would be necessary with cluster sampling as with simple random sampling to obtain the desired level of precision. This specifies that the variance with cluster sampling will be twice as large as the variance with simple random sampling if the same total number, n, of observations were selected with both. It is normally cheaper to sample n observations with cluster sampling than it does with simple random sampling. This is due to the dramatically reduced cost and time involved in constructing sampling frames. This suggests that, for the same cost, one can afford to select many more sampling units, precision is generally greater with cluster sampling. Hence, one would decide how many observations were necessary using the formulae presented in Chapter 8 for simple random sampling.

Example I.8.5
In Example I.8.1 when simple random sampling was used to estimate P to within 5 percentage points with 95% confidence, 338 children would have been needed. If cluster sampling were to be used, how many clusters, and of what size, would be needed for the same precision?

Solution
Assuming a design effect of 2, 676 (i.e. 2 x 338) children would be needed. Some information on the heterogeneity of the clusters and the costs involved would be needed in order to determine the sizes of the clusters. For example the 676 children may be distributed in the following different ways:

Number of clusters	Cluster size
10	68
15	45
20	34
25	27
30	23

The mix of number of clusters (m) and cluster sizes ($\bar{n}$) depends upon the degree of heterogeneity of the clusters. When the variation between clusters is large, we would choose $\bar{n}$ small and m large. Alternatively, the closer the P_i in the clusters are to 0.5, the larger will be the variability within the clusters. In this case, $\bar{n}$ should be large relative to m. Another factor in determining the mix of m and n is cost. The total cost of selecting a cluster sample can be expressed as

$$c = c_1 m + c_2 m \bar{n},$$

where c_1 is the cost involved in selecting clusters (e.g., constructing frames, renting office space, etc.), and c_2 is the cost involved in selecting sampling units (e.g., travel expenses, interviewer expenses, data processing costs). Common sense dictates that if c_1 is large, we would tend to take more sampling units and fewer clusters. However, if c_2 is large, we would take more clusters and fewer sampling units within each cluster.

---

[s] See page 86

Part II
Foundations of Sampling and Statistical Theory

1 The population

The population (or **universe**) is the entire set of individuals for which the findings of a study are to be generalized. The individual members of the population whose characteristics are to be measured are called the **elementary units** or **elements** of the population.

For example, if we are conducting a survey , in a defined area, to determine the proportion of children vaccinated against polio, the universe includes all children living in the area and each child living in that area is an elementary unit.

The primary purpose of almost every sample survey is to *estimate* certain values relating to the distributions of specified characteristics of a population. These values are most often means, totals, proportions or ratios. In this manual, we will concentrate on estimating the **proportion** of individuals possessing a particular characteristic.

Sample surveys belong to a larger class of nonexperimental studies generally given the name "observational studies", which include prospective cohort and retrospective case-control studies. In a cohort study, two or more groups of individuals are identified whose members differ with respect to the presence or absence of a risk factor presumed to be associated with the development of some outcome (for example some disease). All individuals are studied over time to observe whether the incidence of the outcome is higher in the exposed group than it is in the unexposed group. Estimates of the risk of development of disease associated with levels of the risk factor are made through computation of the **relative risk** and its associated confidence interval.

In case-control studies a group of persons with a disease or condition is identified as is a group of individuals without the disease or condition. Individuals in both groups are compared with respect to the presence or absence of characteristics thought to be associated with the disease or condition. Potential risk factors may be identified and estimates of risk are obtained through the computation of the **odds ratio** and its associated confidence interval. Cohort and retrospective case control studies often involve specific **hypotheses** concerning a set of **dependent** (or **response**) variables and another set of **independent** (or **explanatory**) variables. To address these hypotheses, statistical tests may be performed and the hypotheses will be either "rejected" or "not rejected", accordingly.

In contrast to observational studies, an "experimental study" is characterized by the randomization of subjects to "treatments", and the observation of the subject's response to the treatment assigned. Because of the interventional characteristic of experimental studies, the experimenter plays a much more active role than is the case in an observational study. The primary purpose of most experimental studies is to test some research hypothesis. In an experimental study the subjects are usually not representative of the population as a whole. Hence it is typically required that the experiment be repeated in a number of different settings before the results can be thought to apply to a larger, untested group of subjects. A common example of an experimental study is the randomization of patients with a particular condition to one of two groups: (1) an "experimental" group receiving a newly developed pharmaceutical product or (2) a "control" group receiving a placebo or the standard product. Responses in the two "treatment" groups are measured and the hypothesis of equality of response is tested.

Elementary units

The total number of elementary units in the population is denoted in this manual by **N**, and each elementary unit will be identified by a label in the form of a number from 1 to N. A **characteristic** (or **random variable**) will be denoted by an upper case letter, such as Y. The **value of the characteristic** Y in the ith elementary unit will be denoted by Y_i.

Population parameters

The objectives of most sample surveys include estimating the values of certain characteristics of the population from which the sample was selected. These population values are called **parameters**, and for a given population the value of the parameter is constant. Among the most commonly estimated population parameters are the mean and the proportion which may be defined as follows:

Population mean: The population mean of a characteristic X is denoted by "μ" and is computed as:

$$\mu = (\sum_{i=1}^{N} X_i)/N .$$

Population proportion: A population proportion is a population mean for the special situation in which the random variable Y is given by

$$Y_i = 1 \text{ if the attribute Y is present in any element unit i}$$
$$Y_i = 0 \text{ if the attribute Y is not present in any element unit i}$$

Whenever the characteristic being measured represents the presence or absence of some attribute, the variable is said to be dichotomous. In this case, the goal is to estimate the proportion of elementary units in the population having the attribute. If the attribute is denoted by Y, then $\sum_{i=1}^{N} Y_i$ is the total number of elements in the population having the attribute. Let **P** denote the **population proportion** of elements having the attribute where

$$P = (\sum_{i=1}^{N} Y_i)/N .$$

Population variance and **standard deviation**: The variance and the standard deviation of the distribution of a characteristic in a population are important quantities because they measure the *spread* or *dispersion* in the collection of all values. The population variance of a characteristic X is denoted σ^2. Its value is given by the following expression:

$$\sigma^2 = \sum_{i=1}^{N} (X_i - \mu)^2/N .$$

The population standard deviation, denoted by σ, is simply the positive square root of the variance and is given by:

$$\sigma = \sqrt{\left[\sum_{i=1}^{N} (X_i - \mu)^2 / N\right]} .$$

When the characteristic being considered is a dichotomous variable, it can be shown that the population variance as defined above reduces to the following expression:

$$\sigma^2 = NP(1-P).$$

2 The sample

The primary objective of a sample survey is to estimate population parameters using data from a sample.

Probability and nonprobability sampling

Sample surveys can be categorized into two very broad classes on the basis of how the sample was selected, namely, probability samples and nonprobability samples. A **probability sample** has the characteristic that every element in the population has a known probability of being included in the sample. A **nonprobability sample** is one based on a sampling plan which does not incorporate probabilities into the selection process. Examples of nonprobability samples include *quota surveys* (in which interviewers are instructed to contact and interview a specified number of individuals from particular demographic subgroups) and *judgmental samples* (in which the interviewer exercises personal judgment in deciding which sampling units are most representative of the population as a whole and should be included in the sample. In probability sampling, because every element has a known chance of being selected, the reliability of the resulting population estimates can be evaluated objectively through probability theory. Consequently, individuals using the survey estimates have some insight into the reliability of the estimates. In nonprobability sampling, no such insight can be obtained mathematically. Only probability samples will be discussed in this manual.

Sampling frames, sampling units and enumeration units

In probability sampling the probability of any element appearing in the sample must be known. For this to be accomplished, a list must be available from which the sample can be selected. Such a list is called a **sampling frame** and must have the property that every element in the population has some known chance of being included in the sample by whatever method is used to select elements from the sampling frame. A sampling frame does not have to list all elements in a population. For example, if a city directory is used as a sampling frame for a sample survey in which the elements are residents of the city, then clearly all the elements would not be listed in the sampling frame, which in this instance is a listing of households. However, every element has some chance of being selected in the sample if the sampling frame actually enumerates all households in the city.

Often a sampling design specifies that the sampling be performed in two or more stages; such designs are called **multistage sampling designs**. For example, a survey of vaccination coverage in a country might first involve selecting a sample of cities and towns and then, within each of these, selecting a sample of households. In multistage surveys, a different sampling frame is used at each stage of sampling. The units listed in the frame are generally called **sampling units**. In the example above, the sampling frame for the first stage is the list of cities and towns in the country, and each city or town is a sampling unit for this stage. A list of households within each selected city or town constitutes the sampling frame for the second and final stage, and each household is a sampling unit for this stage. The sampling units for the first stage are called **primary sampling units** (PSUs). The sampling units for the final stage of a multistage sampling design are called **enumeration units** or **listing units**.

When conducting a sample survey it is often not convenient to sample the elementary units directly because lists of elementary units from which the sample can be taken are not readily available and cannot be constructed without great difficulty or expense. Fortunately, however, elementary units can often be associated with other kinds of units for which lists can be compiled for the purposes of sampling. These other kinds of units are known as **enumeration units** or **listing units** or **sampling units**. An enumeration unit may contain one or more elementary units and can be identified prior to selecting the sample. For example, in studying vaccination of children in a city, it is unlikely that an accurate and up-to-date list of all children would be available or could be constructed at a reasonable cost prior to sampling. However, it is conceivable that a list of all households is available or at least could be obtained without great difficulty or expense. The households are the enumeration units. If such a list is available, a sample of households can be drawn, and those children residing in the sample households are taken as the elementary units.

Sample measurements and summary statistics

Let us suppose that a sample of n elements has been selected from a population containing N elements and that each sample element is measured with respect to some variable Y. For convenience the sample elements are labeled from 1 to n (no matter what their original labels were in the population). We let y_1 denote the value of Y for the sample element labeled "1"; we let y_2 denote the value of Y for the sample element labeled "2"; and so on. (In general, capital letters such as X and Y will denote a variable and lower case letters such as x and y will denote observed sample values of the variables. In this book a continuous variable is denoted by X and a dichotomous variable by Y.) Having taken the sample, quantities ssuch as means, totals, proportions and standard deviations can be computed, just as for the population. However, when these quantities are calculated for a sample, they are not population parameters since they are subject to sampling variability (a parameter is a constant). These sample values are referred to as **statistics**. Definitions of some statistics that are used later in this book are as follows:

Sample mean: The sample mean with respect to some characteristic X is denoted by $\bar{x}$ and its value is given by the following equation:

$$\bar{x} = \sum_{i=1}^{N} x_i/n .$$

Sample proportion: When the characteristic Y being measured represents presence or absence of some attribute, the sample mean becomes the sample proportion which is denoted by "p". Its value is given by the following equation:

$$p = \sum_{i=1}^{N} y_i/n$$

where the numerator is the number of sample elements having the attribute.

Sample variance and sample standard deviation: For any characteristic X the sample variance is denoted by s^2, and its value is given by

$$s^2 = \sum_{i=1}^{N} (x_i - \bar{x})^2/(n-1).$$

When the characteristic is a dichotomous attribute, the sample variance s^2 as defined above reduces to

$$s^2 = np(1-p)/(n-1) .$$

The sample standard deviation, denoted by s, is simply the positive square root of the sample variance.

Estimates of population characteristics

Estimates of population means and proportions and variances can be obtained directly from the sample means and proportions and variances. An estimate of a population characteristic is denoted by using the symbol $\wedge$ (hat) over the symbol for the population parameter. For example, an estimate of the population proportion is denoted as $\hat{P}$, and the sample proportion is used for this purpose (i.e., $\hat{P} = p$).

With simple random sampling, $\bar{x}$ and s^2 and p as defined above are used to estimate μ, σ^2, and P respectively. These sample statistics ($\bar{x}$, s^2, p) may not always be the correct estimate of the population parameters. For example, if a multistage sample incorporating such features as stratification and clustering was selected from the population, then the correct estimate might have to incorporate statistical weighting factors which reflect the complexity of the sample design used.

Estimates of population parameters obtained from a particular sample can never be assumed to be equal to the true value of the population parameters. If we had taken a different sample, we would have obtained different estimates of these parameters, which may have been either closer or further away from the true parameter values than the estimates from the first sample. Since we never know the true value of the population parameters that we are estimating, we never know how close or how far our sample estimates really are from the true population values. If, however, our sampling plan uses a probability sample, then we can, through mathematics, obtain some insight into how far away from the unknown true values our sample estimates are likely to be. In order to do this, we must know something about the distribution of our estimates. This distribution encompasses all possible samples that can arise from the particular sampling plan being used.

3 Sampling distribution

Suppose that a particular sampling plan and estimation procedure could result in "T" possible samples from a given population and that a particular sample results in an estimate, $\hat{\theta}$, of θ. (The symbol θ here represents any population parameter [e.g., μ, P or σ^2] while the symbol $\hat{\theta}$ represents an estimate of this parameter [e.g., $\bar{x}$, p or s^2]). The collection of values of $\hat{\theta}$ over the T possible samples is called the **sampling distribution** of $\hat{\theta}$ with respect to the specified sampling plan and estimation procedure.

To illustrate a sampling distribution, consider the following simple example.

Example II.3.1
Suppose in a hypothetical district with thirty villages, it is necessary to estimate the proportion of the villages in which less than 50% of the eligible children are immunized against polio. It is decided to randomly select a sample of five villages in which the immunization histories of all the eligible children will be collected to determine the polio immunization levels for each village. This hypothetical population of thirty villages is shown in Table II.1. An indicator Y represents the immunization coverage with a "1" indicating a village with less than 50% of the eligible children immunized against polio, and a "0" indicating immunization level above 50%. (In real life the immunization levels of the villages would of course not be known in advance.)

Table II.1 Data on immunization status in 30 villages

Village	Proportion immunized < 50%	Y	Village	Proportion immunized < 50%	Y
1	yes	1	16	yes	1
2	no	0	17	yes	1
3	yes	1	18	no	0
4	yes	1	19	yes	1
5	yes	1	20	no	0
6	no	0	21	yes	1
7	no	0	22	no	0
8	no	0	23	no	0
9	yes	1	24	yes	1
10	yes	1	25	no	0
11	yes	1	26	no	0
12	yes	1	27	yes	1
13	no	0	28	yes	1
14	yes	1	29	yes	1
15	no	0	30	no	0

If a sampling plan is specified in which five villages are selected at a time at random out of the thirty, such a procedure would yield 142 506 possible samples. Each of these samples has the same chance of being selected. In terms of the notation described in the definition of a sampling distribution, T = 142 506, P=0.57, and each $\hat{\theta}$ = p, where P and p are the population and estimated population proportion, respectively. The sampling distribution of the estimated proportion, p, is given in Table II.2.

Table II.2 Sampling distribution of estimated proportion of samples of size five of the data of Table II.1

p	Frequency	Relative frequency
0.0	1287	0.009
0.2	12155	0.085
0.4	38896	0.273
0.6	53040	0.372
0.8	30940	0.217
1.0	6188	0.043

The relative frequencies shown in the last column of Table II.2 show the fraction of all possible samples that can take on the corresponding values of p. These are shown graphically in Fig. 12.

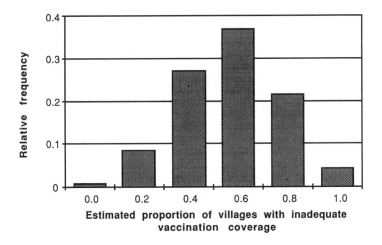

Fig. 12   Relative frequency histogram of sampling distribution of p

Sampling distributions have also certain characteristics associated with them. For our purposes, the two most important of these are the mean and the variance (or its square root, the standard deviation).

The **mean of the sampling distribution** of an estimated parameter $\hat{\theta}$ is also known as its **expected value**, denoted by $E(\hat{\theta})$, and is defined by the equation

$$E(\hat{\theta}) = \sum_{i=1}^{T} \hat{\theta}_i / T$$

where T is the number of possible samples and $\hat{\theta}_i$ is the sample statistic computed from the ith possible sample selected from a population. Note that some of the values of $\hat{\theta}_i$ may be the same from sample to sample, but each one appears in the sum even if there is duplication.

The **variance of the sampling distribution** of an estimated parameter θ, denoted by Var(θ), is defined as

$$\text{Var}(\hat{\theta}) = \sum_{i=1}^{T} [\hat{\theta}_i - E(\hat{\theta})]^2 / T$$

The **standard deviation of the sampling distribution** of an estimated parameter θ is more commonly known as the standard error of θ and is simply the positive square root of the variance Var(θ) of the sampling distribution of θ. This quantity is denoted as

$$SE(\hat{\theta}) = \sqrt{\text{Var}[(\theta)]}.$$

Using these general equations, it is possible to derive expressions for the mean (or expected value), variance and standard error of the sampling distribution of any estimator of interest. In particular, for the sample proportion, assuming simple random sampling of elementary units,

$$E(p) = P$$
$$\text{Var}(p) = P(1-P)/n$$
and
$$SE(p) = \sqrt{\{P(1-P)/n\}}.$$

For the sample mean, x̄, the mean, variance and standard error of the sampling distribution are $E(\bar{x}) = \mu$, $\text{Var}(\bar{x}) = \sigma^2/n$ and $SE(\bar{x}) = \sigma/\sqrt{n}$, respectively.

A very important theorem in statistics which concerns the sampling distributions of sample proportions and means, is known as the **central limit theorem**. This theorem states, in effect, that if the sample means and proportions are based on large enough sample sizes, their sampling distributions tend to be **normal**, irrespective of the underlying distribution of the original observations. (The normal distribution provides the foundation for much of statistical theory. Readers unfamiliar with the normal distribution and its properties would be advised to refer to Dixon and Massey[11] or other basic statistics textbooks.) Hence assuming the sample size is large, the sampling distribution of p may be represented as follows:

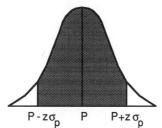

$$P - z\sigma_p \qquad P \qquad P + z\sigma_p$$

Fig. 13 Sampling distribution of p

Here z is the number of standard errors from the mean of the sampling distribution and σ_p= SE(p). How large the sample size (n) must be for the central limit theorem to hold depends on P. For practical purposes, n is sufficiently large if nP is greater than 5. At z equal to 1.96 in Fig. 13, the shaded area under the normal curve equals 95% of the total area. If z=2.58, then the area equals 99%. Using the central limit theorem we can determine how close a sample proportion p is likely to be to the true proportion P in the population from which that sample was selected. This is discussed in greater detail in the following sections.

Two-stage cluster sampling[t]

In the following discussion, we will assume that the same number of listing units are sampled from each cluster selected at the first stage (i.e. $n_i=\bar{n}$, i=1,...,m). To estimate the population proportion, P, we compute

---

[t] See pages 83-86

$$\hat{P} = [M/(Nm)](\sum_{i=1}^{m} N_i \hat{P}_i),$$

where: M = total number of clusters
            m = number of clusters selected at first stage
            N_i = number of sampling units in i^{th} cluster
            N = number of sampling units in the population
            $\hat{P}_i$ = estimate of P_i in i^{th} cluster.

In the above formula,

$N_i \hat{P}_i$ estimates the total number of individuals with the characteristic in the ith cluster;

$\sum_{i=1}^{m} N_i \hat{P}_i$ estimates the total number of individuals with the characteristic over all

m clusters in the sample;

$\sum_{i=1}^{m} N_i \hat{P}_i/m$ estimates the mean number of individuals with the characteristic per

sample cluster;

$M\sum_{i=1}^{m} N_i \hat{P}_i/m$ estimates the total number of individuals with the characteristic in

all M clusters in the population; finally,

$[M/Nm](\sum_{i=1}^{m} N_i \hat{P}_i)$ estimates the proportion of individuals in the population with

the characteristic.

The variance of P is composed of two parts and is expressed as follows:

$$Var(\hat{P}) = M[M-m]/[(M-1)N^2m]\sum_{i=1}^{M}(N_iP_i-NP/M)^2+M/(mN^2)\sum_{i=1}^{M}[N_i^2(N_i-n_i)/(N_i-1)][P_i(1-P_i)/n_i]$$

The first part of this expression represents the variation due to selecting m clusters, primary sampling units (PSU's), from the M available clusters. The second part is the sum of the sampling variation within clusters caused by selecting n_i observations from the N_i which are available.

Since the above expression is a population parameter depending upon knowledge concerning all M population clusters, and true proportions within those clusters, it is necessary to specify an estimate of $Var(\hat{P})$, which may be done as follows:

$$\widehat{Var}(\hat{P}) = [M(M-m)]/[N^2m(m-1)]\sum_{i=1}^{m}\left[N_i\hat{P}_i-(1/m)\sum_{i=1}^{m}N_i\hat{P}_i\right]^2 +$$

$$M/(mN^2)\sum_{i=1}^{m}\{N_i^2[(N_i-n_i)/N_i](1/n_i)[1/(n_i-1)][n_i\hat{P}_i(1-\hat{P}_i)]\}$$

This expression is quite involved, incorporating N_i, n_i and P_i for each of the m clusters selected in the sample. From a sample size determination point of view this is a problem, since different combinations of cluster sample sizes could be used in order to obtain some pre-specified level of precision. A simplified formula may be obtained by specifying that each population cluster be the same size (i.e., $N_i = \bar{N}$) and that the sample size selected from each cluster be the same (i.e., $n_i = \bar{n}$). In that special case, it follows that

$$\hat{Var}(\hat{P}) = (M-m)/[Mm(m-1)]\sum_{i=1}^{m}(\hat{P_i}-\bar{P})^2 + (\bar{N}-n)/[\bar{N}Mm(n-1)]\sum_{i=1}^{m}\hat{P_i}(1-\hat{P_i})$$

where $P = \sum_{i=1}^{m}\hat{P}_i/m$, and $N = M\bar{N}$. Also, $\hat{P}$ becomes

$$\hat{P} = (1/m)\sum_{i=1}^{m}\hat{P}_i = (1/mn)\sum_{i=1}^{m}\sum_{j=1}^{\bar{n}}y_{ij}.$$

The advantage of the above formula is that once M, m and the P_i, i=1,...,m are specified, it would be possible to solve for n, the number of sampling units to select from each cluster. However, it is rather unrealistic to assume that N_i=N for each of the clusters. A more reasonable approach would therefore be to use probability proportionate to size (PPS) cluster sampling. In this strategy, clusters are selected proportional to the number of listing units in the cluster. In this way, clusters with large N_i have a greater chance of being included in the sample than clusters having small N_i. In PPS sampling the same number, n, of listing units is generally sampled from each cluster selected at the first stage. The method is illustrated using the following example.

Example II.3.2

Consider the population of ten villages along with the number of families living in each village, as shown in Table II.3.

Table II.3 Distribution of families in ten hypothetical villages

Villages (clusters)	Number of families, N_i	Cumulative ΣN_i	Random numbers	Random Number chosen
1	4288	4288	00001-04288	04285
2	5036	9324	04289-09324	
3	1178	10502	09325-10502	
4	638	11140	10503-11140	
5	27010	38150	11141-38150	11883;35700;36699
6	1122	39272	38151-39272	
7	2134	41406	39273-41406	
8	1824	43230	41407-43230	
9	4672	47902	43231-47902	
10	2154	50056	47903-50056	

How would a PPS sample of n=4n families be taken?

Solution

We first list these clusters and cumulate the number of listing units (families) as shown in column 3 of Table II.3. Numbers 1 through 4288 are associated with cluster 1; numbers 4289-9324 are associated with cluster 2; numbers 9325 through 10502 are associated with cluster 3; and so on. Four random numbers, between 1 and 50056, 36699, 35700, 11883 and 4285 are selected corresponding to clusters 5, 5, 5 and 1, respectively. For each of the four random numbers chosen, we take a simple random sample of $\bar{n}$ families from the village corresponding to the random number. In this example, three independent simple random samples of $\bar{n}$ families would be selected from village 5 since it corresponds to three of the random numbers, and one simple random sample of $\bar{n}$ families would be selected from village 1.

With PPS cluster sampling, P is estimated by $\hat{P}_{pps}$, where

$$\hat{P}_{pps} = [1/(m\bar{n})]\sum_{i=1}^{m}\sum_{j=1}^{\bar{n}}y_{ij} = (1/m)\sum_{i=1}^{m}\hat{P}_i.$$

It should be noted that the expected value of this estimate is the true population proportion. Hence $\hat{P}_{pps}$ is an **unbiased estimate**[u] of P.

Also, the expression for the estimated variance of $\hat{P}_{pps}$ is

$$\hat{Var}(\hat{P}_{pps}) = \{1/[m(m-1)]\}\sum_{i=1}^{m}(\hat{P}_i-\hat{P}_{pps})^2.$$

Comparing these formulae to the ones presented earlier for non-PPS cluster sampling, one notes that the great advantage of using PPS cluster sampling is the resulting computational simplicity.

The question of sample size is basic to the planning of any cluster sample. Decisions have to be made on, first, the number of clusters, m, which should be selected from the M available clusters and, second, the number of sampling units, $\bar{n}$, which should we select from each cluster. We want to determine m and n so that

$$z_{1-\alpha/2}\sqrt{\hat{Var}(\hat{P}_{pps})} = d.$$

[u] See pages 61-63

4 Characteristics of estimates of population parameters

It would seem intuitively clear that a desirable property of a sampling plan and estimation procedure is that it should yield estimates of population parameters for which the mean of the sampling distribution is equal to, or at least close to, the true unknown population parameter and for which the standard error is very small. In fact, the accuracy of an estimated population parameter is evaluated in terms of these two characteristics.

The **bias** of an estimate $\hat{\theta}$ of a population parameter θ is defined as the difference between the mean, $E(\hat{\theta})$, of the sampling distribution of $\hat{\theta}$ and the true value of the unknown population parameter θ,

$$\text{Bias}(\hat{\theta}) = E(\hat{\theta}) - \theta .$$

An estimate $\hat{\theta}$ is said to be **unbiased** if $\text{Bias}(\hat{\theta}) = 0$, or, in other words, if the mean of the sampling distribution of $\hat{\theta}$ is equal to θ. The sample proportion and sample mean are examples of unbiased estimates when we have random sampling. Recall that the population variance is defined as

$$\sigma^2 = \sum_{i=1}^{N} (X_i - \mu)^2 / N .$$

One estimate of σ^2 might be a similar statistic computed on the n elements selected in the sample. That is,

$$\hat{\sigma}^2 = \sum_{i=1}^{n} (x_i - \bar{x})^2 / n .$$

It can be shown mathematically that

$$E(\hat{\sigma}^2) = [(n-1)/n]\sigma^2 .$$

Hence, $\hat{\sigma}^2$ is a *biased* estimate of σ^2. Alternatively, consider the sample variance presented earlier as

$$s^2 = \sum_{i=1}^{n} (x_i - \bar{x})^2 / (n-1).$$

It can be shown that

$$E(s^2) = \sigma^2 .$$

Hence, s^2 is an *unbiased* estimate of σ^2.

Expected values are based on the *average over all possible samples* which can be selected from a population. In any practical situation, however, the population is likely to be very large and only a single sample is selected from it. It is highly unlikely that the estimate produced from this single sample will exactly equal the population parameter. For this reason, we must define the term "sampling error".

The **sampling error** is the difference between a sample estimate and a population parameter. The population parameter could, in theory, be determined only if a complete study were carried out of every individual in the population of interest. In practice, of course, this is never the case since populations are too large and are constantly changing; as a result, a well-selected sample is the best one can hope for.

To illustrate sampling error, consider the following example.

> **Example II.4.1**
> Suppose the proportion of individuals with hypertension living in a certain community is 0.23. (It should be noted that this proportion is based on a snapshot of the population at an instant in time. Shortly after this snapshot is taken, some members of the population die or move away, while new members arise by birth or in-migration. Hence, defining the population is a more complex issue than may seem at first.) The population parameter is represented as
>
> $$P = 0.23.$$
>
> Suppose a representative sample of the population is studied and the proportion of the sampled individuals with hypertension is 28%. This is denoted by
>
> $$p = 0.28.$$
>
> Using this notation, the sampling error is defined as
>
> $$p - P = 0.28 - 0.23 = 0.05.$$

In this example, the value 0.28 is called a **point estimate**. In general, if θ is some population parameter, and if $\hat{\theta}$ is an estimate of θ, then $\hat{\theta} - \theta$ is the sampling error.

Note that sampling error refers to the relationship between an estimate resulting from a single sample and a population parameter. To account for the existence of sampling error confidence intervals are used rather than point estimates when making statements about population parameters. A confidence interval has the general form:

$$A \leq \theta \leq B$$

and has the following interpretation. Suppose a sample of size n is selected from a population with an unknown parameter θ; the estimate $\hat{\theta}_1$ would not be expected to equal θ exactly . Suppose this process of selecting a sample of size n was performed many times (say "k" times), each sample resulting in a new value of $\hat{\theta}_i$, i=1,...,k. The collection of the k estimates of θ constitutes the sampling distribution which, as a result of the central limit theorem, can be approximated by the normal distribution with mean $E(\hat{\theta})$ and variance $Var(\hat{\theta})$. If the normal distribution adequately describes the sampling distribution, then 95% of all values of $\hat{\theta}$ will fall in the interval:

$$\theta - 1.96\sqrt{Var(\hat{\theta})} \quad \text{to} \quad \theta + 1.96\sqrt{Var(\hat{\theta})}.$$

Only 5% of the time will the estimate $\hat{\theta}$ fall more than $1.96\sqrt{Var(\hat{\theta})}$ units away from the mean, $E(\hat{\theta})$. Since the value of $Var(\hat{\theta})$ is a population parameter, it must be estimated from the sample data. This quantity, denoted by $V\hat{a}r(\hat{\theta})$, is used in the construction of confidence intervals for θ. For example the 95% confidence interval would take the form:

$$\hat{\theta} - 1.96\sqrt{V\hat{a}r(\hat{\theta})} \leq \theta \leq \hat{\theta} + 1.96\sqrt{V\hat{a}r(\hat{\theta})}.$$

The interpretation of this interval is that if confidence intervals such as this were constructed for each of all possible samples which could be selected from a population,

95% of all such intervals would include the true value of θ in the population. Since any particular interval either does or does not cover the mean, the "probability" of a particular interval being correct is either 0 or 1. "Confidence" relates to the theoretical concept of repeatedly sampling from the population. The value of 1.96 implies the inclusion of the central 95% of the area under the normal curve (see Fig. 13). Other choices would be used if different areas were desired (e.g., 2.58 would be used for a 99% confidence interval). For some parameters, such as μ, the t-distribution rather than the normal distribution, would be used for the purpose of describing the confidence interval if the variance was estimated from the data and if the sample size was small. (Readers unfamiliar with the t-distribution and its properties should refer to an appropriate basic textbook of statistics.) The following example illustrates the construction of a confidence interval for a population proportion.

Example II.4.2
In order to estimate the proportion of children in a particular school vaccinated against polio, a list of all students is assembled and a simple random sample of 25 of these students is selected. The proportion of students in the sample vaccinated against polio is observed to be 44%. The 95% confidence interval estimate of P, the true proportion vaccinated in the school, is

$$0.44 - 1.96\sqrt{[0.44(1-0.44)/25]} \leq P \leq 0.44 + 1.96\sqrt{[0.44(1-0.44)/25]}$$
or
$$0.25 \leq P \leq 0.63.$$

This states that if confidence intervals of this type were established for all possible random samples of size 25 which could be selected from this population, 95% of these would correctly incorporate the true proportion vaccinated in the population. The interval 0.23 to 0.62 either does or does not include the true P so in that sense, the "probability" of it being correct is either 0 or 1. We have "confidence" in this interval because of our knowledge of the nature of the sampling distribution as well as how such intervals perform upon repeated sampling. (Since the population proportion P is unknown, p(1-p) is used as an estimate of the variance of the sampling distribution, P(1-P).)

Precision relates to the confidence interval and is defined in terms of repeated sampling. That is,

$$\text{precision} = [\text{reliability coefficient}] \times [\text{standard error}]$$

where the reliability coefficient reflects the desired confidence and is represented by a z-value if normality is assumed. For example, if the desired confidence is 95%, then the reliability coefficient is the upper 97.5th percentile of the normal distribution with mean 0, and variance 1. This is represented by $z_{0.975}$.

5 Hypothesis testing

In the above discussion, our primary aim was estimating the unknown population parameter. We now consider the situation where there is an underlying hypothesis which is to be tested. A **null hypothesis** (H_0) is simply a statement concerning the value of the population parameter. For example, the statement might be that the proportion of pregnant women receiving adequate prenatal care in a particular city is 80%. This may be stated in notational form as:

$$H_0: P = 0.8.$$

The statistician considers this statement as a possibility and, based on a knowledge of the sampling distribution, decides which values of the sample statistic (in this case the sample proportion, p) could reasonably be expected to occur if the hypothesized value was, in fact, the actual population parameter. From the previous discussion regarding sampling distributions we know that if a large number of random samples were selected from a population, the sample statistic θ would fall in the interval between $\theta+1.96\sqrt{Var(\theta)}$ and $\theta-1.96\sqrt{Var(\theta)}$ 95% of the time. Hence, any value of θ which falls in this interval would not be considered an unlikely result of a random sample from the population with parameter θ. However, any value of θ beyond 1.96 standard errors from θ would be considered an unlikely event if the population parameter was, in fact, θ.

Every null hypothesis has an associated alternative. The **alternative hypothesis** is a statement of what the value of the parameter is in the population if the null hypothesis is not correct. The alternative hypothesis is denoted H_a. For example, if the null hypothesis is that the population proportion is 0.8, the alternative could be that the population proportion is something other than 0.8. This would be stated as

$$H_0: P = 0.8$$

versus

$$H_a: P \neq 0.8.$$

This particular statistical hypothesis H_0, is compared to a **two-sided alternative** since the null hypothesis is rejected if the value of the sample proportion is either too large or too small. A **one-sided alternative** is one in which the null hypothesis is rejected if the observed value of the statistic differs significantly from the hypothesized parameter in one direction. For example, the null hypothesis might be that the proportion of pregnant women in the population receiving adequate prenatal care is 0.80 and an intensified program would be initiated if it can be demonstrated that the true proportion is *less than* 80%. That is,

$$H_0: P = 0.8$$

versus

$$H_a: P < 0.8.$$

In this case, rejection of the null hypothesis in favor of H_a calls for action. Failure to reject H_0 would provide no evidence to suggest that the level of prenatal care in the community is inadequate and no immediate action would be called for. The **rejection region** for the test specifies, *in advance of selecting the sample*, those values of p which would result in the rejection of the null hypothesis. If the sample yields a value of p which is not in the rejection region, the appropriate conclusion is that there is no evidence to reject H_0. The null hypothesis is never "accepted" since a sample resulting in a particular value of p could have been selected from many populations, and it is impossible to know exactly which one it was.

A **type I (or alpha [α]) error** occurs whenever a null hypothesis which is true is incorrectly rejected. The probability of making this type of error may be controlled by the investigator and is denoted by α. This may be expressed by the following notation:

$$\alpha = \text{Prob\{committing a type I error\}} = \text{Prob\{rejecting } H_0 | H_0 \text{ is true\}} .$$

Because of our understanding of the nature of the sampling distribution, the size of the α-error may be controlled by the investigator. For example, since it is known that only 5% of sample proportions will differ from the true population proportion by more than 1.96 standard errors, a rejection region composed of all sample proportions above and below 1.96 standard errors from the mean would have an α-error of 5%. That is, 5% of all possible samples which could be selected from a population would result in sample proportions either above $P+1.96\sigma_p$ or below $P-1.96\sigma_p$.

On the other hand, if the null hypothesis is not rejected, there is a chance that it was, in fact, false and should have been rejected. This type of error is termed the **type II (or beta [β]) error**. The probability of making a type II-error is denoted β.

$$\beta = \text{Prob\{committing a type II error\}} = \text{Prob\{failing to reject } H_0 | H_0 \text{ is false\}} .$$

Finally, the **power of the test** is defined as the probability of correctly rejecting H_0 given H_0 is false. That is,

$$\textbf{1-}\beta = \text{Power} = \text{Prob\{rejecting } H_0 | H_0 \text{ is false\}}.$$

These concepts can be summarized in the following figure.

		Actual population	
		H_0 is true	H_0 is false
Decision	Fail to reject H_0	$1 - \alpha$	β Type II error
	Reject H_0	α Type I error	$1 - \beta$ Power

Fig. 14 Summary of the probabilities of the possible outcomes in hypothesis testing

From Fig. 14 we see that in any given hypothesis test only one type of error can be committed. That is, if we reject H_0 only an α-error could be made if H_0 were actually true. On the other hand, if we fail to reject H_0 we could be inadvertently committing a β error if H_0 were actually false.

Figs 15 and 16 depict these concepts for a two-sided and a one-sided test respectively. In Fig. 15, a statistical test is being performed concerning a population proportion. Under H_0, the population proportion equals P_0 while under H_a, the population proportion differs from P_0. That is

$$H_0: P=P_0 \text{ versus } H_a: P \neq P_0 .$$

Since it is not known whether the true P in the population is actually above or below P_0, Fig. 15 shows the situation in which it is assumed that $P_a > P_0$. A similar figure could have been drawn for $P_a < P_0$.

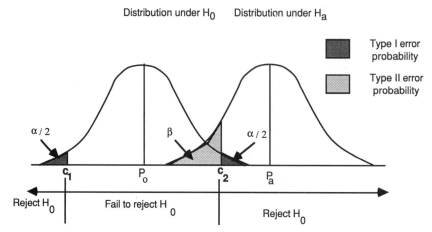

Fig. 15 Two-sided test of the population proportion

Fig. 16 depicts a test of $H_0: P = P_0$ versus $H_a: P < P_0$.

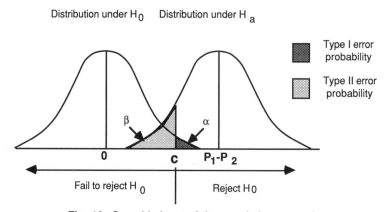

Fig. 16 One-sided test of the population proportion

As seen in Figs 15 and 16, the probability of making a type II error and the power of the test vary according to the true P; the further the true P is from P_0, the smaller the type II error (and the larger the power). In determining the sample size a suitable combination of P_a and β is fixed together with the level of α. The way this is done is described in Part I.

Example II.5.1

Suppose that as a method for screening a community to determine prenatal care levels, 50 births are to be randomly selected and use of prenatal care by the mother is assessed. If the results were to indicate that less than 80% of the mothers had received "adequate" prenatal care then some appropriate action would be initiated in the community. Suppose that 32 of the 50 mothers selected are judged to have received "adequate" prenatal care, what conclusions can be made about prenatal care in the community?

Solution

A one-sided rejection region is implied since action is to be taken only if the level of care is *less than* 80%.

Therefore: H_0: $P = 0.80$ versus H_a: $P < 0.80$

Under the null hypothesis, and invoking the central limit theorem, the sampling distribution of the sample proportion is normal with:

$$
\begin{aligned}
\text{mean} \quad &= 0.80 \\
\text{standard error} \quad &= \sqrt{[(0.80 \times 0.20/50)]} \\
&= 0.0566
\end{aligned}
$$

 (Note that 1.645 is the z-value corresponding to the number of standard errors to the left of the mean of a normal distribution such that only 5% of the area under the curve will be smaller.)   Hence the decision rule is to reject the null hypothesis if the sample proportion is less than:

$$0.80 - 1.645 \times 0.0566 = 0.707$$

Since $p = 32/50 = 0.64$, the null hypothesis of "adequate" prenatal care should be rejected. A corrective appropriate action should therefore be initiated.

6 Two-sample confidence intervals and hypothesis tests

So far all attention has focused on the situation where a single sample has been selected from some population and we either estimated or tested a hypothesis concerning a parameter in the population. Now suppose that interest focuses on determining whether the populations from which two samples were selected have the same parameter.

As an example, suppose all women of childbearing age seeking contraception in Community A are supplied with one type of contraceptive while all women in Community B are supplied with a second type of contraceptive. It is of interest to determine whether the proportion of unplanned pregnancies among women in Community A is equivalent to the proportion in Community B. In this example the first population is of all women who could ever be given the first contraceptive while the second population is of all women who could ever be given the second contraceptive. The women in Community A are considered to be a sample from this first population while the women in Community B are considered to be a sample from the second population.

If both populations have the same parameter the statistical question is whether or not the difference observed between the two sample statistics could be due to chance alone. This question can be addressed either through the establishment of a confidence interval or by testing an appropriate null hypothesis.

The difference between the two sample values is also a statistic. If sets of two samples were repeatedly selected and the difference between the sample values was calculated, the set of differences would constitute a new sampling distribution - the sampling distribution of the difference. The mean of this sampling distribution is:

$$E(\hat{\theta}_1 - \hat{\theta}_2) = 0$$

and, assuming the two samples are *independent*, the variance of this distribution is

$$Var(\hat{\theta}_1 - \hat{\theta}_2) = Var(\hat{\theta}_1) + Var(\hat{\theta}_2).$$

As a specific example, if the study is designed to test H_0: $P_1=P_2$ then the mean of the sampling distribution of p_1-p_2 under H_0 is 0 and the variance is:

$$Var(p_1-p_2) = Var(p_1) + Var(p_2) = P_1(1-P_1)/n_1 + P_2(1-P_2)/n_2$$

where n_1 and n_2 are the number of observations selected from the first and second samples. If the null hypothesis is true, $P_1=P_2=P$. Hence it follows that

$$Var(p_1-p_2) = P(1-P)/n_1 + P(1-P)/n_2 = P(1-P)(1/n_1+1/n_2)$$

and if the sample sizes are equal, i.e., $n_1=n_2=n$, then

$$Var(p_1-p_2) = 2[P(1-P)/n].$$

This variance involves the unknown population parameter, P. As a result, this parameter is usually estimated by the average of the two sample proportions. That is, assuming $n_1=n_2=n$,

$$\hat{P} = \bar{P} = (p_1+p_2)/2.$$

Fig. 17 presents the two-sample hypothesis testing situation for proportions.

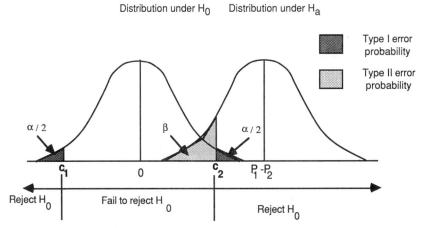

Fig. 17 Two-sample, two-sided test of H_0: $P_1=P_2$ vs H_a: $P_1 \neq P_2$

Example II.6.1
Suppose two drugs are available for the treatment of a particular type of intestinal parasite. One hundred patients entering a clinic for treatment for this parasite are randomized to one of the two drugs; fifty receiving drug A and fifty receiving drug B. Of the patients receiving drug A, 64% responded favorably; 82% of the patients receiving drug B responded favorably. Are the drugs equally effective or is the observed difference too large to be due to chance alone?

Solution
The problem is set up assuming the two drugs are equally effective and, so long as there is no economic or other reason to prefer one drug over the other, the test can be set up two-sided. That is,

$$H_0: P_1=P_2 \text{ or } H_0: P_1-P_2=0$$
$$H_a: P_1 \neq P_2 \text{ or } H_a: P_1-P_2 \neq 0$$

Our decision rule, at the 5% level of significance, is to reject H_0 if p_1-p_2 is greater than $0+1.96\sqrt{[2(0.73)(0.27)/50]} = 0.174$ or less than $0-1.96\sqrt{[2(0.73)(0.27)/50]} = -0.174$. The value 0.73 is the average of the proportions responding in each group (previously denoted p). In the actual trial, $p_1-p_2 = 0.64-0.82 = -0.18$. Therefore, since this falls in the rejection region (i.e., $-0.18 < -0.174$), the null hypothesis is rejected in favor of the alternative that the drugs are not equally effective.

An alternative approach for testing this hypothesis is to first establish a confidence interval whose end points are given in the following expression:

$$(p_1-p_2) \pm z_{1-\alpha/2}\sqrt{[p_1(1-p_1)/n_1+p_2(1-p_2)/n_2]}$$

and then determine whether or not the value 0, i.e., the value which would indicate no difference between the population proportions, falls in the interval. If it does, the null hypothesis is not rejected; if it does not, the null hypothesis is rejected.

Example II.6.2
In Example II.6.1, the end points of the confidence interval are:

$$(0.64-0.82)\pm1.96\sqrt{[(0.64)(0.36)/50 + (0.82)(0.18)/50]}$$

$$-0.18 \pm 1.96(0.0869) = -0.18 \pm 0.17,$$

yielding the 95% confidence interval,

$$-0.35 \leq P_1 - P_2 \leq -0.01.$$

Notice that 0 does not fall in this interval so that again we would conclude, using a confidence interval approach, that the two drugs are not equally effective.

Note that when establishing a confidence interval the sample proportions are not pooled to obtain an estimate of the variance of the difference since there is no underlying null hypothesis stating that the population parameters are equal.

Confidence intervals have a major advantage over hypothesis tests - more information is obtained about the population parameter than the simple rejection or acceptance of a statement. When testing a null hypothesis we always run a risk of committing an error. The type-I or α error is possible whenever the null hypothesis is rejected. Fortunately, the magnitude of this error probability is fixed and may be stated in advance by the investigator. Whenever the hypothesis cannot be rejected, there exists the possibility of committing a type-II or β error. It is unfortunately true that one never knows how large the β error is since one never knows the actual condition of the population.

7 Epidemiologic study designs

Earlier discussion concerning the two group problem has centered on either estimating the true difference between the proportions in the two groups or on testing the hypothesis that the proportions in the populations from which the samples were selected are equal. That discussion was presented within the context of the **cohort** or **follow-up** study. The key element in the cohort study is that individuals are grouped according to whether or not they have a certain characteristic which is suspected to be related to the outcome of interest. This characteristic will be called the **exposure** variable. Individuals in the various exposure groups (usually presence and absence of exposure) are subsequently followed until a determination of the **outcome** characteristic (e.g., disease or no disease) can be made. For the epidemiologist, however, this type of study design may not be practical when the time between exposure and outcome is lengthy and/or unknown. For example, a cohort study to assess the relationship between consumption of artificial sweeteners and bladder cancer would not be practical for at least two major reasons. First, in order to obtain a sufficiently large group of patients who develop the disease, a huge sample would have to be identified when they are disease-free and then followed for several years to determine subsequent disease status. This is due to the fact that the disease is relatively rare. Second, because exposure is at relatively low levels, a long exposure time would be necessary before the disease could be expected to develop. This presents numerous logistical problems, not the least of which is keeping track of and staying in contact with a large number of study subjects for a long period of time. Finally, from a practical point of view, if sweeteners are suspected of being associated with bladder cancer, we would not want to wait twenty years or so to have confirmatory scientific evidence. Hence, a cohort design is not a realistic option for many modern epidemiologic investigations on chronic diseases.

In a **case-control** design, subjects are selected on the basis of their outcome status (e.g. patients with bladder cancer are enlisted into the study, as is a group of "controls" or non-cancer patients) and all subjects are studied with respect to their prior and current exposure to suspected risk factors. From a practical point of view, this type of study may be carried out at relatively low cost and within a relatively short time frame since it is not necessary to wait for the disease to develop in previously disease-free individuals.

There is a third type of epidemiologic study known as a **prevalence study**. In this type of study, a representative sample is selected from the population in order to estimate the proportion of individuals with a condition of interest at a specific point in time. This condition can relate to either exposure or to disease and is typically presented as a proportion. This proportion is termed the **prevalence** and represents an instantaneous snapshot of the number of people with the condition at a specified point in time relative to the total number of eligible individuals in the population. The concept of prevalence is distinct from that of **incidence** which is a measure of the number of new cases occurring in the population in a specified time period. Prevalence may be either greater than or less than incidence depending upon the duration of the condition and the rate at which incident cases die or leave the population. Hence one measure cannot be substituted for the other.

The relative risk and odds ratio

Central to understanding the importance of the cohort and case-control studies in epidemiologic research designs are the parameters **relative risk** and **odds ratio**. Table II.4 presents the tabular display which will be used in the discussion of these concepts. In this table, D and $\bar{D}$ represent the presence and absence of disease, respectively. Similarly, E and $\bar{E}$ represent exposure and nonexposure to the suspected risk factor.

Table II.3　Tabular display of disease/exposure relationship

E x p o s u r e

D i s e a s e	Present (E)	Absent ($\bar{E}$)	Total
Present (D)	a	b	n_1
Absent ($\bar{D}$)	c	d	n_2
Total	m_1	m_2	n

In the cohort study, n individuals are enrolled in the study. All of these individuals are disease-free at the beginning of the study and n_1 of them are known to be subsequently exposed to a suspected risk factor while n_2 of them are not.

The relative risk, denoted "RR", is a population parameter defined as the ratio of the probability of disease development among exposed individuals to the probability of disease development among nonexposed individuals. The expression Prob{A|B} will denote the probability of the event "A" among all individuals having the characteristic "B". Using this notation, the relative risk is:

$$RR = \text{Prob}\{D|E\}/\text{Prob}\{D|\bar{E}\}.$$

This parameter may be estimated **directly** only in a cohort study since in that type of study the outcome, presence or absence of disease, is the measured variable. In fact, Prob{D|E} and Prob{D|$\bar{E}$} may be estimated by a/n_1 and c/n_2 respectively. Thus, the relative risk may be estimated as

$$\hat{RR} = (a/m_1)/(b/m_2)$$

The remarkable feature of a case-control study is that it permits estimation of the relative risk under certain conditions. This is accomplished via the **odds ratio**. The **odds of an event** is defined as the ratio of the probability that the event will occur to the probability that the event will not occur. For example, in the **cohort study**, let the odds in the exposed group be denoted as "O_1" where

$$O_1 = \text{Prob}\{D|E\}/\text{Prob}\{\bar{D}|E\}.$$

Let the odds in the unexposed group be denoted as "O_2" where

$$O_2 = \text{Prob}\{D|\bar{E}\}/\text{Prob}\{\bar{D}|\bar{E}\}.$$

As its name implies, the **odds ratio**, denoted by "OR", is the ratio of O_1 to O_2. That is,

$$OR = O_1/O_2.$$

From Table II.4 it is clear that to estimate the odds ratio for a cohort study we compute

$$OR = [(a/m_1)/(c/m_1)]/[(b/m_2)/(d/m_2)] = ad/bc.$$

In a *case-control study*, the measured variable is the exposure status of the individual. Thus, for the cases, the odds is defined as $\text{Prob}\{E|D\}/\text{Prob}\{\bar{E}|D\}$ while, for the controls, the odds is given by $\text{Prob}\{E|\bar{D}\}/\text{Prob}\{\bar{E}|\bar{D}\}$. Hence, the odds ratio for case-control studies is

$$OR = [\text{Prob}\{E|D\}/\text{Prob}\{\bar{E}|D\}]/[\text{Prob}\{E|\bar{D}\}/\text{Prob}\{\bar{E}|\bar{D}\}].$$

From Table II.4 it can be seen that to estimate this quantity from a case-control study we compute

$$\hat{OR} = [(a/n_1)/(b/n_1)]/[(c/n_2)/(d/n_2)] = ad/bc.$$

The quantity ad/bc is also called the **cross product ratio** in the literature of 2x2 contingency tables. We see that the odds ratio, as estimated by the cohort study, is identical to the odds ratio as estimated by the case-control study. While odds ratios may be estimated from either case-control or cohort studies, relative risks may only be estimated directly from cohort studies.

In many, if not all, epidemiologic studies, the parameter of primary interest is the relative risk, RR, since this parameter quantifies how much more (or less) likely an individual who has been exposed is to develop the outcome than is an individual who has not been exposed. In the epidemiologic literature, relative risks of order of magnitude 2 (providing they are statistically significant) or larger are often considered important evidence of an exposure effect.

In many epidemiologic studies the diseases being studied are relatively rare events and, as a result, $\text{Prob}\{D|E\}$ and $\text{Prob}\{D|\bar{E}\}$ are both small. The relative risk, as estimated from a cohort study, is

$$
\begin{aligned}
\hat{RR} &= (a/m_1)/(b/m_2) \\
&= [a/(a+c)]/[b/(b+d)] \\
&= (ab+ad)/(ab+bc) \\
&= (ad/bc)\{[(b/d)+1]/[(a/c)+1]\} \\
&= \hat{OR}\,\{[(b/d)+1]/[(a/c)+1]\}
\end{aligned}
$$

If the odds ratio is used as an estimate of the relative risk, the expression $\{[(b/d)+1]/[(a/c)+1]\}$ should be approximately one - which will be the case if b/d and a/c are small. This will be true if the number of individuals without the disease is very large relative to the number of individuals with the disease in both the exposed and unexposed groups. Thus when the disease is rare, we may approximate the value of the relative risk by the value of the odds ratio which in turn may be estimated from the case-control study design.

In the previous discussion of hypothesis testing and estimation of proportions the notation P_1 and P_2 were used to denote the proportions with the condition in populations 1 and 2 respectively. Putting this into the framework of the cohort study, where the subscript 1 denotes the exposed cohort and the subscript 2 denotes the unexposed cohort, it follows that

$$P_1 = \text{Prob}\{D|E\}, \quad 1-P_1 = \text{Prob}\{\bar{D}|E\}$$

$$P_2 = \text{Prob}\{D|\bar{E}\}, \quad 1-P_2 = \text{Prob}\{\bar{D}|\bar{E}\}$$

For the case-control study, similar notation may be defined for the probabilities of exposure given disease presence or absence. That is, define

$$P_1{}^* = \text{Prob}\{E|D\}, \quad 1-P_1{}^* = \text{Prob}\{\overline{E}|D\}$$

$$P_2{}^* = \text{Prob}\{E|\overline{D}\}, \quad 1-P_2{}^* = \text{Prob}\{\overline{E}|\overline{D}\}.$$

It follows that

$$RR = P_1/P_2$$

and that

$$OR = [P_1{}^*/(1-P_1{}^*)]/[P_2{}^*/(1-P_2{}^*)].$$

In terms of the notation of the 2x2 table in Table II.4 the parameters may be estimated as follows:

$$p_1 = a/m_1, \quad 1-p_1 = c/m_1$$

$$p_2 = b/m_2, \quad 1-p_2 = d/m_2$$

$$p_1{}^* = a/n_1, \quad 1-p_1{}^* = b/n_1$$

$$p_2{}^* = c/n_2, \quad 1-p_2{}^* = d/n_2$$

Estimates of the relative risk and odds ratio may be defined as:

$$\hat{RR} = p_1/p_2 = (a/m_1)/(b/m_2) = am_2/bm_1$$

$$\hat{OR} = [p_1{}^*/(1-p_1{}^*)]/[p_2{}^*/(1-p_2{}^*)] = ad/bc.$$

The sampling distribution of the odds ratio

Because the odds ratio, OR, may take on values between 0 and ∞, with a value of 1 indicating no excess risk, it follows that the sampling distribution of the estimated odds ratio will tend to be nonnormal, exhibiting strong positive skewness (i.e., a longer tail to the right). For skewed distributions such as this, the $\log_e$ (natural logarithm denoted by "ln") transformation will often improve the distributional properties, making the distribution much more normal in shape. As a result, the most commonly employed large-sample method for determining a confidence interval estimate for the odds ratio, or for testing hypotheses about the odds ratio, is to do all calculations based on ln(OR). Confidence limits determined on logarithmic scale may then be transformed to the original scale by exponentiation. That is:

$$e^{\ln(OR)} = OR.$$

Following exponentiation of the limits, the resulting confidence interval will not be symmetric, the direction of the skew depending upon whether the odds ratio ($\hat{OR}$) was greater or less than one.

It follows, from statistical methods for determining the variance of a function of a random variable, that the variance of the sampling distribution of $\ln(\hat{OR})$ is approximately

$$\text{Var}[\ln(\hat{OR})] = (1/n_1)\{ 1/[P_1{}^*(1-P_1{}^*)] \} + (1/n_2)\{1/[P_2{}^*(1-P_2{}^*)] \}$$

Since this expression involves unknown population parameters, an estimate of this quantity may be obtained as

$$\text{Vâr}[\ln(\hat{OR})] = 1/a + 1/b + 1/c + 1/d .$$

Fig. 18 shows the use of ln(OR) and the relationship between the confidence limits as defined on the two scales.

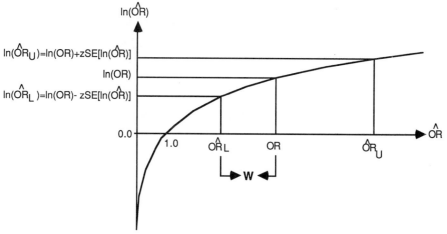

Fig. 18 Plot of confidence interval for ln(OR) versus confidence interval for OR

Fig. 18 shows that, whereas the confidence interval established for ln(OR) is symmetric, when the limits are transformed into the original scale the transformed interval is not symmetric about OR.

If a statistical test of the null hypothesis $H_0{:}OR=1$ versus the alternative $H_a{:}OR{\neq}1$ is to be performed, the usual chi-square (χ^2) test based on the 2x2 table may be used. If the resulting calculated value of χ^2 is too large, the null hypothesis is rejected. (The previously described test of the equality of two proportions is equivalent to this chi square test based on the 2x2 table.)

To illustrate these concepts, consider the following example.

Example II.7.1
Thirty patients with cancer have been identified along with 150 controls who were in the hospital at the same time but for other conditions. Twenty-four of the cancer patients smoke while 90 of the non-cancer patients smoke. The data layout is as follows:

Smoking

Cancer status	Yes	No	Total
Yes	24	6	30
No	90	60	150
Total	114	66	180

For these data the estimated odds ratio is $(24)(60)/[(90)(6)] = 2.67$. To determine whether 2.67 is significantly different from 1, test the hypothesis $H_0:OR=1$ versus $H_a:OR \neq 1$, by computing the usual chi-square test with one degree of freedom. Here, $\chi^2=4.31$ which is significant at the 5% level. [Note that the critical region is reject H_0 if $\chi^2 > \chi^2_{1-\alpha}(1)$.] Hence we reject H_0.

A confidence interval estimate for the population odds ratio is obtained by first taking the $\log_e$ of the estimated odds ratio, utilizing the standard error of the $\ln(OR)$ to construct a confidence interval for $\ln(OR)$, and finally exponentiating to obtain a confidence interval for the odds ratio. In this example, the log odds is $\ln(2.67)=0.981$. The estimated variance of the log odds is:

$$Var[\ln(OR)]=1/24+1/90+1/6+1/60 = 0.236.$$

The 95% confidence interval for $\ln(OR)$ is:

$$0.981 - 1.96\sqrt{0.236} \leq \ln(OR) \leq 0.981 + 1.96\sqrt{0.236}$$

$$0.029 \leq \ln(OR) \leq 1.93$$

Converting to original units it follows that

$$e^{0.029} \leq OR \leq e^{1.93}$$

$$1.03 \leq OR \leq 6.9 .$$

Since 1 does not fall in this interval, we again see that we would reject H_0. This may not always be the case since the chi-square test and the method for confidence interval estimation are based on different distributional assumptions: (p_1-p_2) and $\ln(OR)$, respectively. The reader should see Fleiss[17] for a complete discussion of the various methods for estimation and testing of the odds ratio.

The literature on estimation and hypothesis testing about odds ratios is very large and most attention has focused on the situation where n_1, n_2, m_1 and m_2 (see Table II.4), are small. Since the goal of this manual is sample size determination, and since these sample sizes will tend to be large, the methods based on $\ln(\hat{OR})$ will be appropriate.

The sampling distribution of $\hat{RR}$ will, for extremely large samples, be approximated by a normal distribution. However, for sample sizes typically employed in most epidemiologic studies, the sampling distribution of $\hat{RR}$ will often not be normal, with considerable skewness to the right (as was the case with $\hat{OR}$). A logarithmic transformation is again employed which induces more symmetry into the sampling distribution, allowing use of the normal distribution to approximate the sampling distribution for smaller sample sizes. Thus, as was the case with the odds ratio, confidence interval estimation of the RR is usually performed by first obtaining a confidence interval for $\ln(RR)$ and later exponentiating the confidence limits to obtain a confidence interval for the RR parameter.

Recall that the relative risk is estimated from a cohort study as

$$\hat{RR} = p_1/p_2$$

and it follows, from standard methods used to obtain the variance of a function of a random variable, that:

$$Var[\ln(\hat{RR})] = Var[\ln(p_1)-\ln(p_2)] = Var[\ln(p_1)] + Var[\ln(p_2)] .$$

Now, since the variance of the $\log_e$ of any proportion p based on n observations is

$$Var[\ln(p)] = (1/n)[(1-P)/P]$$

it follows that the variance may be estimated as

$$\hat{Var}[\ln(\hat{RR})] = (1/m_1)[(1-p_1)/p_1] + (1/m_2)[(1-p_2)/p_2].$$

This expression for the estimate of the variance of the $\log_e$ of the relative risk is then used in precisely the same way as was the expression for the variance of the odds ratio for construction of confidence intervals. Again, the limits of the symmetric confidence interval for the ln(RR) must be exponentiated in order to obtain a confidence interval for the relative risk. This interval will not be symmetric, as was illustrated in Fig. 18 for OR.

Screening tests for disease prevalence

In any given population, certain individuals have a specified disease while others do not. For example, we know that at any particular point in time, there are some women in a population who have cervical cancer while the vast majority of women do not. Early detection of this disease is vital for assuring a favorable prognosis. The PAP test has been advocated as a screening device for detecting prevalent cancerous or pre-cancerous lesions.

No screening test is 100% accurate. That is, it is possible that a patient with the disease will not be identified by the screening test. Alternatively, it is possible that a disease-free patient could have a positive result on the screening test. A framework for thinking about these types of errors can be established in the following way:

We will hypothesize that the patient has the disease. If we reject H_0, we will conclude that the patient is disease free; otherwise, we will continue to assume the patient has the disease and will undergo the next level of screening (e.g., the patient with a positive PAP test might then have a punch biopsy to verify the initial result).

That is,
        H_0: Patient has cervical cancer
versus
        H_a: Patient does not have cervical cancer

We will base our decision on a single screening test (PAP test) which will be used as a diagnostic tool for early detection of cervical cancer. It is important to set up the screening test such that the alternative is the disease-free condition. This allows one to take advantage of the size of the type I error. By this we mean that if we reject H_0, the only type of error which could have occurred is a type I error, which we may make as small as we wish.

Consider the 2x2 table presented in Fig. 19 which relates to the decisions made on a number of patients:

True condition of patient

Fig. 19   Classification table of true condition versus decision

Fig. 19 shows that a total of n patients have been screened. Of these, $n_1.$ had a positive result and $n_2.$ had a negative result. Furthermore, we assume that all n patients were studied in detail following the screening and $n._1$ were determined to actually have the disease while $n._2$ were determined to be free of the disease. Using these data, we may estimate numerous quantities of interest.

True positive rate = $n_{11}/n._1$ - This rate is also called the **sensitivity** of the test.

False negative rate = $n_{21}/n._1$ - This rate is equivalent to the α error of the hypothesis test.

False positive rate = $n_{12}/n._2$ - This rate is equivalent to the β error of the hypothesis test.

True negative rate = $n_{22}/n._2$ - This rate is also called the **specificity** of the test. It is equivalent to the statistical power of the hypothesis test.

It should be noted that in any actual study, the values of $n._1$ and $n._2$ would not be known. Instead, we may be interested in the **predictive values**. These may be estimated as follows:

Predictive value of a positive = $n_{11}/n_1.$ - This is the proportion of individuals with positive screening tests who actually have the disease.

Predictive value of a negative = $n_{22}/n_2.$ - This is the proportion of individuals with negative screening tests who are actually disease free.

The predictive value observed in any study depends upon the prevalence of the disease. If the population being screened is a high risk population, there will be high prevalence and the predictive value of a positive test will be higher than with a low risk population.

8 Basic sampling concepts

This section contains a brief review of the basic strategies used for sampling from human populations. It is intended to serve as a point of reference for the sample size discussions found in the manual. Readers interested in a more detailed discussion are referred to the books on sampling theory.

Because populations tend to be large and resources and time available for studies limited, it is usually not possible to study each elementary unit or each listing unit comprising a population. For this reason there is little choice but to select a sample from the population and then make estimates regarding the entire population. In order for such estimates to be made, it is necessary that some scientifically valid sampling methodology be employed. In the following discussion, the most commonly employed sampling schemes are briefly reviewed.

Simple random sampling

Fig. 20 presents a diagram of a population of N enumeration units.

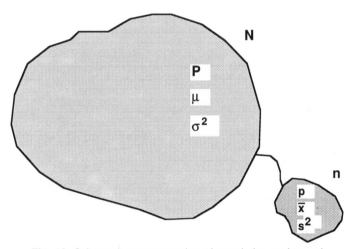

Fig. 20 Schematic representation of population and sample

The proportion of these enumeration units which possess some characteristic, Y, is denoted **P**, the mean level of some characteristic, X, over all N enumeration units is denoted μ, and the variance of the N values of X is denoted σ^2. Because N may be very large or the time or budget available to carry out the survey very limited, a sample of size "n" of the original N enumeration units in the population must be selected. From the n selected enumeration units in the sample, the population proportion, mean and variance may be estimated by p, $\bar{x}$ and s^2. If this sample is selected at random from the population, these estimates will be "unbiased". That is,

$$E(p) = P$$

$$E(\bar{x}) = \mu$$

$$E(s^2) = \sigma^2.$$

From the discussion of Chapter 4 of the second part of this book, this means that if many (e.g., "k") random samples were selected from this population, and if p, x̄ and s^2 were computed for each of these samples, the average of the k sample proportions would equal the population proportion, P, the average of the k sample means would equal μ and the average of the k sample variances would be σ^2. Unbiasedness is a desirable statistical property since it assures that the sample values will, on average, be correct. However, it must be stressed that an estimate computed from any one particular sample may be quite different from the population parameter. The concept of unbiasedness relates to repeated sampling and the corresponding averaging process.

In order to select a simple random sample it is necessary to:

*   Construct a list (or "frame") of the N enumeration units;

*   Use a random process (e.g., a random number table) to generate n numbers between 1 and N which identifies the n individuals in the sample.

Note that there are ^NC_n possible samples which can be selected from this population [where $^NC_n=N!/n!(N-n)!$ and a!=(a)·(a-1)·(a-2)·...·(1)]. For example, if N=25 and a sample of size n=5 is to be selected, there are $^{25}C_5 = 53130$ possible samples. A simple random sample may then be formally defined as follows:

Definition: A *simple random sample* is one in which each of the ^NC_n possible samples has the same chance of being selected; i.e., $1/(^NC_n)$.

The advantages of simple random sampling may be stated as follows:

*   It is simple to conceptualize;

*   It provides the probabalistic foundation of much of statistical theory;

*   It provides a baseline to which other methods can be compared.

The disadvantages of simple random sampling may be listed as follows:

*   All N enumeration units in the population must be identified and labelled prior to sampling. This process is potentially so expensive and time consuming that it becomes unrealistic to implement in practice;

*   Sampled individuals may be highly dispersed. This suggests that visiting each of the sampled individuals may be a very time consuming and expensive process;

*   Certain subgroups in the population may, by chance, be totally overlooked in the sample.

However, because of its several disadvantages, alternatives to simple random sampling are often employed in actual surveys of human populations. The alternative methods may provide more precise estimates (i.e., narrower confidence intervals) for the same cost.

Systematic sampling

This method can save much time and effort and is more efficient in some situations than simple random sampling. For example, suppose a sample, size n, of patients' records, treated during the past year at a local health clinic, is needed for a survey of nutritional intake. With systematic sampling, this is accomplished by creating n zones of k = N/n records each. Within the first zone, a random number between 1 and k is selected, representing the first chosen record. Subsequent records are identified by successively adding the constant k to the starting random number i. Thus, the sample of size n is composed of the ith, $[i+k]^{th}$,...,$[i+(n-1)k]^{th}$ records in the filing cabinet. This is represented pictorially as follows:

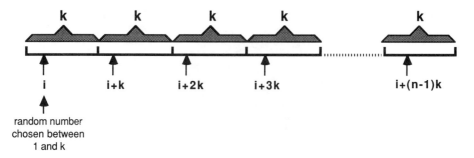

random number
chosen between
1 and k

The advantages of using systematic sampling over simple random sampling may be summarized as follows:

• It may be possible to select a systematic sample in situations where a simple random sample cannot be selected. For example, suppose an audit of hospital records is required on an ongoing basis. In this situation a simple random sample is not possible since N is not known in advance. However, if N can be approximated and if we know what size n is required, a "1 in k" sample can be selected where k=N/n;

• Using systematic sampling the selected sampling units are likely to be more uniformly spread over the whole population and may therefore be more representative than a simple random sample;

• Under most conditions, simple random sampling formulae for parameter and variance estimates can be used with systematic sampling.

Unfortunately, there are some situations where selection of a systematic sample is ill-advised. For example, if the list or frame is arranged in a cyclical fashion and k is the length of the cycle, a highly biased estimate will result. For example, suppose a study of visits to a hospital emergency room is planned. If the emergency room has Sundays as the busiest day of the week while Wednesdays are the least busy, then the cycle is of length 7. If zones of length 7 are established, very unfortunate results may arise as seen in the following diagram.

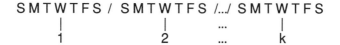

Here, selecting a random number between 1 and 7 resulted in a 4, identifying Wednesday. Then repeatedly adding 7 to this random start results in the selection of successive Wednesdays, the least busy day of the week. Estimates produced from this sample will certainly not be representative of the emergency room's experience. Establishing a zone size which differs from the cycle size effectively eliminates this problem.

Even when cycles do not exist, systematic sampling is often not the method of choice for actual field surveys. This is due to the fact that many of the problems listed previously with simple random sampling apply to systematic sampling as well, and it is possible to get better precision at lower cost with other methods than is possible with systematic sampling.

Stratified sampling

Consider a study of all hospital beds in a particular geographic region. This population is represented pictorially in Fig. 21 as follows:

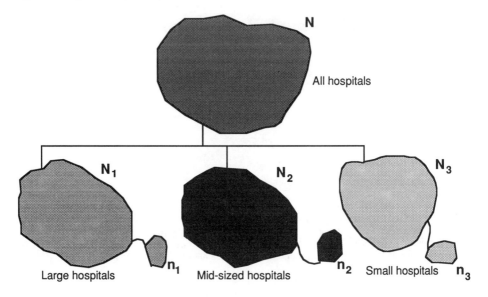

Fig. 21 Schematic representation of stratified sampling

If a simple random sample were selected from the N hospitals, the large hospitals could, by chance alone, be either totally missed, oversampled or undersampled.

Definition: A *stratum* is a subpopulation of the original population. The strata are formed on the basis of some known characteristic about the population which is believed to be related to the variable of interest.

In the hospital example, strata of hospitals may be formed based on number of beds, number of physicians, etc.

Definition: *Stratified random sampling* is the process of breaking down the population into mutually exclusive and exhaustive strata, selecting a random sample from each of the strata, and finally combining these into a single sample to estimate the population parameters.

In order to obtain the highest precision, elements within the strata should be as homogeneous as possible, while stratum-to-stratum variation should be relatively large.

Once it is decided to use stratified random sampling, a decision must be reached as to how many elements are to be selected from each stratum. This is known as **allocation** of the sample. The simplest allocation scheme involves selecting an equal number of observations from each stratum. That is, $n_h = n/L$, where L is the total number of strata, and n_h is the number of elements selected from stratum h. The most commonly utilized allocation scheme is **proportional allocation**. In this scheme, the sampling fraction, n_h/N_h, is specified to be the same for each stratum. That is, the number of elements taken from the hth stratum is given by

$$n_h = (N_h)(n/N) \ .$$

When proportional allocation is used, estimates of the population mean and proportion are "self-weighting". This means that when estimating the population mean, proportion or total, each sample element is multiplied by the same constant, $1/n$, irrespective of the stratum to which the element belongs.

The advantages of stratified random sampling may be summarized as follows:

- A stratified random sample may provide increased precision (i.e., narrower confidence intervals) over that which is possible with a simple random sample of the same size;

- Information concerning estimates within each stratum is easily obtainable;

- For either administrative or logistical reasons, it may be easier to select a stratified sample than a simple random sample.

The major disadvantage of stratified sampling is, however, that it is no less expensive than simple random sampling since detailed frames must be constructed for each stratum **prior to sampling**. For this reason, despite the high level of precision possible with stratified sampling, the most commonly employed sampling method in survey research is cluster sampling.

Cluster sampling

Suppose a survey is being planned to study the prenatal care received by pregnant women in a large city.

Among the numerous problems inherent in such a study are:

- The population is very large and it might be impossible to construct an up-to-date and accurate frame. Even if one could be set up, the costs involved in setting up a detailed frame and later in attempting to contact individuals may be prohibitive;

- The population is highly dispersed. This presents significant logistical problems if there are restrictions on available time and travel expenses.

A solution to these problems is to use a cluster sampling strategy.

Sampling techniques such as simple random sampling and systematic sampling require that the sampling frames be constructed which list the individual enumeration units (or listing units).

Sometimes, however, especially in surveys of human populations, it is not feasible to compile sampling frames of all enumeration units for the entire population. On the other hand, sampling frames can often be constructed that identify **groups** or **clusters** of enumeration units without listing explicitly the individual enumeration units.

Sampling can be performed from such frames by:

- taking a sample of clusters;

- obtaining a list of enumeration units only for those clusters which have been selected in the sample;

- selecting a sample of enumeration units.

Cluster sampling is a hierarchical kind of sampling in which the elementary units are at least one step removed from the original sampling clusters, and often two steps (or more) are involved.

The term "cluster", when used in sample survey methodology, can be defined as any sampling unit with which one or more listing units can be associated. This unit can be geographic or temporal in nature.

Definition: *Cluster sampling* can be defined as any sampling plan that uses a frame consisting of clusters of enumeration units. Typically, the population is divided into "M" mutually exclusive and exhaustive clusters. Unlike strata, clusters should be as **heterogeneous** as possible.

The process by which a sample of listing units is selected is typically stepwise. For example, if city blocks are clusters and households are listing units, there might be two steps involved in selecting the sample households:

• **Step 1**: Select a sample of blocks;

• **Step 2**: Select a sample of households within each block selected at the first step.

Diagrammatically, this may be represented as in Fig. 22 :

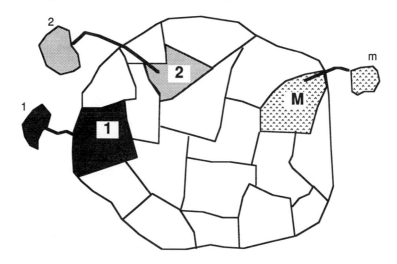

Fig. 22 Schematic representation of cluster sampling

In sampling terminology, these steps are called "stages", and sampling plans are often categorized in terms of the number of stages involved. For example, a "single-stage cluster sample" is one in which the sampling is done in only one step - i.e., once the sample of clusters is selected, every enumeration unit within each of the selected clusters is included in the sample. At the first stage, "m" clusters are selected from the M available clusters. At the second stage, all N_j listing units are studied in the jth selected cluster.

For a "two-stage sample" the "m" clusters are selected from the M available clusters at the first stage. At the second stage, n_j elementary units are selected, using simple random or systematic sampling techniques, from the jth cluster, $j=1,...,m$. Hence samples of size $n_1,n_2,...,n_m$ are selected from the $N_1,N_2,...,N_m$ elementary units comprising the frames of each of the selected clusters.

Note that $n=n_1+n_2+...+n_m$. If $n_i = N_i$, $i=1,...,m$, we have a "simple one-stage cluster sample". On the other hand, if $n_i < N_i$ for some i, we have a two-stage cluster sample.

A "multistage cluster sample" is performed in two or more steps. For example, to carry out an immunization survey of school children in a given province, the following steps might be followed:

- **Step 1**: Select m counties from the M mutually exclusive and exhaustive counties composing the province;

- **Step 2**: Select a sample of townships or other minor civil divisions within each of the counties selected at the first step;

- **Step 3**: Select a sample of school districts within each of the townships selected at the second stage;

- **Step 4**: Select a sample of schools within each of the school districts selected at the third stage;

- **Step 5**: Select a sample of classrooms within each of the schools selected at the fourth stage;

- **Step 6**: Take every child within the classrooms selected at the fifth stage.

In this example, the children are the "elementary units" and the classrooms are the "listing units". In sampling involving more than two stages, the clusters used at the first stage of sampling are generally referred to as "primary sampling units" or "PSUs".

With these multistaged designs, writing down precise expressions for parameter estimates and associated standard errors can be difficult since each level of sampling must be accounted for. Variance estimation techniques such as *jackknife, bootstrap, balanced repeated replication* and *linearization* are invaluable in these circumstances.

It should be noted that in the cluster sampling schemes described thus far, the m clusters were selected **at random** from the M available clusters. (Without loss of generalizability, this selection may be done systematically as well.) When clusters are selected with "probability proportionate to size", denoted "PPS", selection is not random. This method of selection has, however, a number of distinct advantages[24].

The advantage of cluster sampling is that detailed frames need only be constructed for the m clusters selected at the next-to-last stage. This represents great savings in time and resources since frames need not be prepared for the entire population.

Cluster sampling generally will not produce as precise estimates as will simple random sampling or stratified sampling if each method were to use the same total sample size, n. However, due to the greatly reduced cost and administrative ease, a larger cluster sample may be selected, for the same cost, than that which is possible using the other sampling schemes discussed thus far. As a result of the larger sample size, a relatively high level of precision will result.

The two most important reasons why cluster sampling is so widely used in practice, especially in sample surveys of human populations and in sample surveys covering large geographic areas, are **feasibility** and **economy**. Cluster sampling may be the only feasible method since the only frames readily available for the target population may be lists of clusters. If that is the case, it is almost never feasible, in terms of time and resources, to compile a list of individuals (or even households) for the sole purpose of conducting a survey. However, lists of blocks or other geographic units can be compiled relatively easily, and these can serve as the sampling frame of clusters. Cluster sampling is also often the most economical form of sampling since listing costs and travel costs are the lowest of any potential method.

In general, if $n_1=n_2=\cdots=n_m=n$, standard errors obtained by cluster sampling are approximately $\sqrt{\{1+\delta_x(n-1)\}}$ times as large as those obtained from a simple random sample of the same total number of listing units, where δ_x is the intraclass correlation coefficient and n is the number of listing units selected in each cluster. This coefficient δ_x can range from very small negative values, when the elements within each cluster tend to be very diverse or representative of the population of elements (this is termed "heterogeneity"), to a maximum of one when the elements within each cluster are similar but differ from cluster to cluster (this is termed "homogeneity"). It is clear that standard errors with cluster sampling will equal those with simple random sampling when $\delta_x=0$ (i.e., heterogeneous clusters), but can be much larger when the clusters are homogeneous. The ratio of the variance with cluster sampling to the variance with simple random sampling is termed the **design effect**.

Bibliography

Area of emphasis

1. Armitage P: *Sequential Medical Trials*. New York, Halstead Press, 1975. 8

2. Bloch DA: Sample size requirements and the cost of a randomized clinical trial with repeated measurements. *Stat in Med* 5: 663-667, 1986. 3

3. Bohning D: Confidence interval estimation of a rate and the choice of sample size. *Stat in Med* 7: 865-875, 1988. 1,3

4. Browne RH: Reducing sample sizes when comparing experimental and control groups. *Arch Environ Health* May/June: 169-170, 1976. 2,4

5. Brownlee KA: *Statistical Theory and Methodology in Science and Engineering* (2nd ed.). New York, John Wiley & Sons, 1965. 5

6. Casagrande JT, Pike MC, Smith PG: An improved approximate formula for calculating sample sizes for comparing two binomial distributions. *Biometrics* 34: 483-486, 1978. 2

7. Chase G, Klauber MR: A graph of sample sizes for retrospective studies. *Am J Pub Health* 55: 1993-1996, 1965. 2,4

8. Connett JE, Smith JA, McHugh RB: Sample size and power for pair-matched case control studies. *Stat in Med* 6: 53-59, 1987. 2,4

9. Connor RJ: Sample size for testing differences in proportions for the paired-sample design. *Biometrics* 43: 207-211, 1987. 2

10. Daniel WW: *Biostatistics: A Foundation for Analysis in the Health Sciences* (3rd ed.). New York, John Wiley & Sons, 1983. 1,2,7

11. Dixon WJ, Massey FJ: *Introduction to Statistical Analysis* (3rd ed.). New York, McGraw-Hill Book Company, 1969. 1,2,8

12. Donner A: Approaches to sample size estimation in the design of clinical trials--a review. *Stat in Med* 3: 199-214, 1984. 2,3,6

13. Donner A, Birkett N, Buck C: Randomization by cluster-sample size requirements and analysis. *Am J Epidemiol* 114: 906-914, 1981. 7

14. Donner A, Eliasziw M: Sample size requirements for reliability studies. *Stat in Med* 6: 441-448, 1987. 1

15. Feigl P: A graphical aid for determining sample size when comparing two independent proportions. *Biometrics* 34: 111-122, 1978. 2

16. Feinstein AR: XXXIV. The other side of 'statistical significance': alpha, beta, delta, and the calculation of sample size. *Clinical Biostatistics* 18: 491-505, 1975. 2

17. Fleiss JL: Confidence intervals for the odds ratio in case-control studies: the state of the art. *J Chron Dis*, 32: 69-77, 1979. 2,4

The *Area of emphasis* column refers to that part of the reference of particular interest (see Key)

Key
1   One sample
2   Two samples
3   Cohort studies
4   Case-control studies
5   Lot quality assurance sampling
6   Incidence density studies
7   Survey sampling
8   Sequential analysis

18. Fleiss JL: *Statistical Methods for Rates and Proportions* (2nd ed.). New York,
     John Wiley & Sons, 1981.   1,2

19. Fleiss JL, Tytun A, Ury HK: A simple approximation for calculating sample
     size for comparing independent proportions. *Biometrics* 36: 343-346, 1980.   2

20. Freiman JA, Chalmers TC, Smith HS Jr., Kuebler RR: The importance of beta,
     the Type II error and sample size in the design and interpretation of the
     randomized control trial. *NEJM* 299: 690-694, 1978.   2,3

21. Gail M: The determination of sample sizes for trials involving several
     independent 2 x 2 tables. *J Chron Dis* 26: 669-673, 1973.   2,3

22. Gail M, Gart JJ: The determination of sample sizes for use with the exact
     conditional test in 2 x 2 comparative trials. *Biometrics* 29: 441-448, 1973.   2,3

23. George SL, Desu MM: Planning the size and duration of a clinical trial studying
     the time to some critical event. *J Chron Dis* 27: 15-24, 1977.   8

24. Gillum RF, Williams PT, Sondik E: Some considerations for the planning of
     total-community prevention trials - when is sample size adequate?
     J Comm Health 5: 270-278, 1980.   8

25. Greenland S: On sample-size and power calculations for studies using confidence   1,3
     intervals. *Am J Epidemiol* 128: 231-237, 1988.

26. Gross AJ, Clark VA: *Survival Distributions: Reliability Applications in the
     Biomedical Sciences*. New York, John Wiley & Sons, 1975.   6

27. Haber M: Sample sizes for the exact test of 'no interaction' in 2 x 2 x 2 tables.
     Biometrics 39: 493-498, 1983.   2,3

28. Haines T, Shannon H: Sample size in occupational mortality studies.
     J Occup Med 25: 603-608, 1983.   2,3,8

29. Hall JC: A method for the rapid assessment of sample size in dietary studies.
     Am J Clinical Nutrition 37: 473-477, 1983.   2,3

30. Heilbrun LK, McGee DL: Sample size determination for the comparison of   2,3
     normal means when one sample is fixed. *Comp Stat & Data Analysis* 3: 99-102, 1985.

31. Hornick CW, Overall JE: Evaluation of three sample size formulae for 2 x 2
     contingency tables. *J Educ Stat* 5: 351-362, 1980.   2

32. Hsieh FY: A simple method of sample size calculation for unequal-sample-size   2
     designs that use the logrank or t-test. *Stat in Med* 6: 577-581, 1987.

33. Johnson AF: Sample size: clues, hints or suggestions. *J Chron Dis* 38: 721-725, 1985.   3

34. Kalbfleisch JD, Prentice RL: *The Statistical Analysis of Failure Time Data*.
     New York, John Wiley & Sons, 1980.   6

35. Lachenbruch PA: A note on sample size computation for testing interactions.   3
     Stat in Med 7: 467-469, 1988.

36. Lachin JM: Sample size determinations for r x c comparative trials.
     Biometrics 33: 315-324, 1977.   2,3

The *Area of emphasis* column refers to that part of the reference of particular interest (see Key)

Key
1	One sample	5	Lot quality assurance sampling
2	Two samples	6	Incidence density studies
3	Cohort studies	7	Survey sampling
4	Case-control studies	8	Sequential analysis

37. Lachin JM: Introduction to sample size determination and power
    analysis for clinical trials. *Controlled Clinical Trials* 2: 93-113, 1981.   2,6

38. Laird NM, Weinstein MC, Stason WB: Sample-size estimation: a sensitivity
    analysis in the contest of a clinical trial for treatment of mild hypertension.
    Am J Epidemiol 109: 408-419, 1979.   2,3

39. Lee ET: *Statistical Methods for Survival Data Analysis*. Belmont,
    Lifetime Learning Publications, 1980.   6

40. Lemeshow S, Hosmer DW, Klar J: Sample size requirements forstudies estimating   3,4
    odds ratios or relative risks. *Stat in Med* 7: 759-764, 1988.

41. Lemeshow S, Hosmer DW, Stewart JP: A comparison of sample size determination
    methods in the two group trial where the underlying disease is rare.
    Commun Statist Simula Computa, Bio (5): 437-449, 1981.   2

42. Levy PS, Lemeshow S: *Sampling for Health Professionals*.
    Belmont, Lifetime Learning Publications, 1980.   7

43. Likes J: Sample size for the estimation of means of normal populations.
    Biometrics   : 846-849, 1967.   2

44. Lubin JH, Gail MH, Ershow AG: Sample size and power for case-control studies   4
    when exposures are continuous. *Stat in Med* 7: 363-376, 1988.

45. Lwanga SK, Lemeshow S: *Sample Size Determination in Health Studies: A User's Manual.*   1-7
    World Health Organization, Geneva, 1989.

46. Makuch R, Simon R: Sample size requirements for evaluating a conservative
    therapy. *Cancer Treat Rep* 62: 1037-1040, 1978.   2,3

47. Makuch RW, Simon RM: Sample size considerations for non-randomized
    comparative studies. *J Chron Dis* 33: 175-181, 1980.   2,3

48. Makuch RW, Simon RM: Sample size requirements for comparing time-to-failure
    among k treatment groups. *J Chron Dis* 35: 861-867, 1982.   7

49. McKeown-Eyssen G: Sample size determination in case-control studies.   4
    J Chron Dis 40: 1141-1143, 1987.

50. Meydrech EF, Kupper LL: Cost considerations and sample size requirements in
    cohort and case-control studies. *Am J Epidemiol* 107: 201-205, 1978.   2,3,4

51. Miller AT: *Probability and Mathematical Statistics: Applied Probability
    and Statistics*. John Wiley & Sons, New York, 1981.   6

52. Moss S, Draper GJ, Hardcastle JD, Chamberlain J: Calculation of sample size in   3
    trials of screening for early diagnosis of disease. *Int J Epidemiol* 16: 104-110, 1987.

53. Mullooly JP: Sample sizes for estimation of exposure-specific disease rates in   4
    population-based case-control studies. *Am J Epidemiol* 125: 1079-1084, 1987.

54. Nam J-M: Optimum sample sizes for the comparison of the control and
    treatment. *Biometrics* 20: 101-108, 1973.   2,3

55. Odeh RE, Fox M: *Sample Size Choice; Charts for Experiments with Linear Models*.
    New York, Marcel Dekker, Inc., 1975.   1,2

The *Area of emphasis* column refers to that part of the reference of particular interest (see Key)

Key
1	One sample	5	Lot quality assurance sampling
2	Two samples	6	Incidence density studies
3	Cohort studies	7	Survey sampling
4	Case-control studies	8	Sequential analysis

56. Oliphant TH, McHugh RB: Least significant relative risk determination in the case of unequal sample sizes. *Am J Epidemiol* 113: 711-715, 1981.   2,3,4

57. Overall JE: Sample size required to observe at least k rare events. *Psych Rep* 21: 70-72, 1967.   1

58. Overall JE, Dalal SN: Empirical formulae for estimating appropriate sample sizes for analysis of variance designs. *Perceptual and Motor Skills* 27: 363-367, 1968.   2

59. Palta M: Determining the required accrual rate for fixed-duration clinical trials. *J Chron Dis* 35: 73-77, 1982.   2,8

60. Palta M, McHugh R: Adjusting for losses to follow-up in sample size determination for cohort studies. *J Chron Dis* 32: 315-326, 1979.   2,3,8

61. Pasternack BS, Shore RE: Sample sizes for group sequential cohort and case-control study designs. *Am J Epidemiol* 113: 182-191, 1981.   2,3,4,8

62. Pasternack BS, Shore RE: Sample sizes for individually matched case-control studies. *Am J Epidemiol* 115: 778-784, 1982.   2,4

63. Pocock SJ: *Clinical Trials, a Practical Approach*. Chichester, John Wiley & Sons, 1983.   2

64. Radhakrishna S: Computation of sample size for comparing two proportions. *Indian J Med Res* 77: 915-919, 1983.   2

65. Rao BR: Sample size determination in case-control studies: the influence of the distribution of exposure. *J Chron Dis* 39: 941-943, 1986.   4

66. Rubenstein LV, Gail MH, Santner TJ: Planning the duration of a comparative clinical trial with loss to follow-up and a period of continued observation. *J Chron Dis* 34: 469-479, 1981.   2,8

67. Scheaffer RL, Mendenhall W, Ott L: *Elementary Survey Sampling* (2nd ed.). North Scituate, Duxbury Press, 1979.   1,8

68. Schlesselman JJ: Sample size requirements in cohort and case-control studies of disease. *Am J Epidemiol* 99: 381-384, 1974.   2,3,4

69. Schoenfeld DA: Sample-size formula for the proportional- hazards regression model. *Biometrics* 39: 499-503, 1983.   6

70. Schumacher M: Power and sample size determination in survival time studies with special regard to the censoring mechanism. *Meth Inform Med* 20: 110-115, 1981.   8

71. Takizawa T: Nomograms for obtaining a necessary, minimum sample size: I. When distribution of data is normal. *Nat Inst Anim Hlth Quart* 16: 25-30, 1976.   1

72. Taulbee JD, Symons MJ: Sample size and duration for cohort studies of survival time with covariables. *Biometrics* 39: 351-360, 1983.   2,3,7

73. Tygstrup N, Lachin JM, Juhl E: *The Randomized Clinical Trial and Therapeutic Decisions*. Vol. 43, Statistics: Textbooks and Monographs. New York, Marcel Dekker, Inc., 1982.   2,7

74. United States American Public Health Association: On the use of sampling in the field of public health. *Am J Pub Hlth* 44: 719-740, 1954.   7

The *Area of emphasis* column refers to that part of the reference of particular interest (see Key)

Key

1	One sample	5	Lot quality assurance sampling
2	Two samples	6	Incidence density studies
3	Cohort studies	7	Survey sampling
4	Case-control studies	8	Sequential analysis

75. Ury HK, Fleiss JL: On approximate sample sizes for comparing two independent proportions with the use of Yates' correction. *Biometrics* 36: 347-351, 1980.　　2

76. Wetherill GB: *Sequential Methods in Statistics.* New York: John Wiley & Sons, 1966.　　8

77. Wu M, Fisher M, DeMets D: Sample sizes for long-term medical trial with time-dependent dropout and event rates. *Controlled Clinical Trials* 1: 109-121, 1980.　　2,3,7

78. Yamane T: *Elementary Sampling Theory.* Englewood Cliffs, Prentice-Hall, Inc., 1967.　　1,7

79. Young MJ, Bresnitz EA, Strom BL: Sample size nomograms for interpreting negative clinical studies. *Annals Intern Med* 99: 248-251, 1983.　　2,3

The *Area of emphasis* column refers to that part of the reference of particular interest (see Key)

Key

1	One sample	5	Lot quality assurance sampling
2	Two samples	6	Incidence density studies
3	Cohort studies	7	Survey sampling
4	Case-control studies	8	Sequential analysis

Part III
Tables for Sample Size Determination

Table 1a: Sample Size Necessary to Estimate **P** to Within **d** Absolute Percentage Points with **99%** Confidence

Anticipated Population Proportion (P)

d	0.05	0.10	0.15	0.20	0.25	0.30	0.35	0.40	0.45	0.50	0.55	0.60	0.65	0.70	0.75	0.80	0.85	0.90	0.95
0.01	3152	5972	8461	10617	12442	13935	15096	15926	16424	16589	16424	15926	15096	13935	12442	10617	8461	5972	3152
0.02	788	1493	2115	2654	3111	3484	3774	3981	4106	4147	4106	3981	3774	3484	3111	2654	2115	1493	788
0.03	350	664	940	1180	1382	1548	1677	1770	1825	1843	1825	1770	1677	1548	1382	1180	940	664	350
0.04	197	373	529	664	778	871	944	995	1026	1037	1026	995	944	871	778	664	529	373	197
0.05	126	239	338	425	498	557	604	637	657	664	657	637	604	557	498	425	338	239	126
0.06	88	166	235	295	346	387	419	442	456	461	456	442	419	387	346	295	235	166	88
0.07	64	122	173	217	254	284	308	325	335	339	335	325	308	284	254	217	173	122	64
0.08	49	93	132	166	194	218	236	249	257	259	257	249	236	218	194	166	132	93	49
0.09	39	74	104	131	154	172	186	197	203	205	203	197	186	172	154	131	104	74	39
0.10	32	60	85	106	124	139	151	159	164	166	164	159	151	139	124	106	85	60	32
0.11	26	49	70	88	103	115	125	132	136	137	136	132	125	115	103	88	70	49	26
0.12	22	41	59	74	86	97	105	111	114	115	114	111	105	97	86	74	59	41	22
0.13	19	35	50	63	74	82	89	94	97	98	97	94	89	82	74	63	50	35	19
0.14	16	30	43	54	63	71	77	81	84	85	84	81	77	71	63	54	43	30	16
0.15	14	27	38	47	55	62	67	71	73	74	73	71	67	62	55	47	38	27	14
0.20	8	15	21	27	31	35	38	40	41	41	41	40	38	35	31	27	21	15	8
0.25	5	10	14	17	20	22	24	25	26	27	26	25	24	22	20	17	14	10	5

Table 1b: Sample Size to Estimate P to Within **d** Absolute Percentage Points with **95%** Confidence

Anticipated Population Proportion (**P**)

d	0.05	0.10	0.15	0.20	0.25	0.30	0.35	0.40	0.45	0.50	0.55	0.60	0.65	0.70	0.75	0.80	0.85	0.90	0.95
0.01	1825	3457	4898	6147	7203	8067	8740	9220	9508	9604	9508	9220	8740	8067	7203	6147	4898	3457	1825
0.02	456	864	1225	1537	1801	2017	2185	2305	2377	2401	2377	2305	2185	2017	1801	1537	1225	864	456
0.03	203	384	544	683	800	896	971	1024	1056	1067	1056	1024	971	896	800	683	544	384	203
0.04	114	216	306	384	450	504	546	576	594	600	594	576	504	504	450	384	306	216	114
0.05	73	138	196	246	288	323	350	369	380	384	380	369	350	323	288	246	196	138	73
0.06	51	96	136	171	200	224	243	256	264	267	264	256	243	224	200	171	136	96	51
0.07	37	71	100	125	147	165	178	188	194	196	194	188	178	165	147	125	100	71	37
0.08	29	54	77	96	113	126	137	144	149	150	149	144	137	126	113	96	77	54	29
0.09	23	43	60	76	89	100	108	114	117	119	117	114	108	100	89	76	60	43	23
0.10	18	35	49	61	72	81	87	92	95	96	95	92	87	81	72	61	49	35	18
0.11	15	29	40	51	60	67	72	76	79	79	79	76	72	67	60	51	40	29	15
0.12	13	24	34	43	50	56	61	64	66	67	66	64	61	56	50	43	34	24	13
0.13	11	20	29	36	43	48	52	55	56	57	56	55	52	48	43	36	29	20	11
0.14	9	18	25	31	37	41	45	47	49	49	49	47	45	41	37	31	25	18	9
0.15	8	15	22	27	32	36	39	41	42	43	42	41	39	36	32	27	22	15	8
0.20	5	9	12	15	18	20	22	23	24	24	24	23	22	20	18	15	12	9	5
0.25	*	6	8	10	12	13	14	15	15	15	15	15	14	13	12	10	8	6	*

* Sample size less than 5

Table 1c: Sample Size to Estimate P to Within d Absolute Percentage Points with **90%** Confidence

Anticipated Population Proportion (P)

d	0.05	0.10	0.15	0.20	0.25	0.30	0.35	0.40	0.45	0.50	0.55	0.60	0.65	0.70	0.75	0.80	0.85	0.90	0.95
0.01	1285	2435	3450	4330	5074	5683	6156	6494	6697	6765	6697	6494	6156	5683	5074	4330	3450	2435	1285
0.02	321	609	863	1082	1268	1421	1539	1624	1674	1691	1674	1624	1539	1421	1268	1082	863	609	321
0.03	143	271	383	481	564	631	684	722	744	752	744	722	684	631	564	481	383	271	143
0.04	80	152	216	271	317	355	385	406	419	423	419	406	385	355	317	271	216	152	80
0.05	51	97	138	173	203	227	246	260	268	271	268	260	246	227	203	173	138	97	51
0.06	36	68	96	120	141	158	171	180	186	188	186	180	171	158	141	120	96	68	36
0.07	26	50	70	88	104	116	126	133	137	138	137	133	126	116	104	88	70	50	26
0.08	20	38	54	68	79	89	96	101	105	106	105	101	96	89	79	68	54	38	20
0.09	16	30	43	53	63	70	76	80	83	84	83	80	76	70	63	53	43	30	16
0.10	13	24	35	43	51	57	62	65	67	68	67	65	62	57	51	43	35	24	13
0.11	11	20	29	36	42	47	51	54	55	56	55	54	51	47	42	36	29	20	11
0.12	9	17	24	30	35	39	43	45	47	47	47	45	43	39	35	30	24	17	9
0.13	8	14	20	26	30	34	36	38	40	40	40	38	36	34	30	26	20	14	8
0.14	7	12	18	22	26	29	31	33	34	35	34	33	31	29	26	22	18	12	7
0.15	6	11	15	19	23	25	27	29	30	30	30	29	27	25	23	19	15	11	6
0.20	*	6	9	11	13	14	15	16	17	17	17	16	15	14	13	11	9	6	*
0.25	*	*	6	7	8	9	10	10	11	11	11	10	10	9	8	7	6	*	*

* Sample size less than 5

Table 2a: Sample Size to Estimate P to Within ε Relative Percentage Points with **99%** Confidence

Anticipated Population Proportion (**P**)

ε	0.05	0.10	0.15	0.20	0.25	0.30	0.35	0.40	0.45	0.50	0.55	0.60	0.65	0.70	0.75	0.80	0.85	0.90	0.95
0.01	1260798	597220	376027	265431	199073	154835	123236	99537	81104	66358	54293	44239	35731	28439	22119	16589	11710	7373	3493
0.02	315200	149305	94007	66358	49769	38709	30809	24885	20276	16590	13574	11060	8933	7110	5530	4148	2928	1844	874
0.03	140089	66358	41781	29493	22120	17204	13693	11060	9012	7374	6033	4916	3971	3160	2458	1844	1302	820	389
0.04	78800	37327	23502	16590	12443	9678	7703	6222	5069	4148	3394	2765	2234	1778	1383	1037	732	461	219
0.05	50432	23889	15042	10618	7963	6194	4930	3982	3245	2655	2172	1770	1430	1138	885	664	469	295	140
0.06	35023	16590	10446	7374	5530	4301	3424	2765	2253	1844	1509	1229	993	790	615	461	326	205	98
0.07	25731	12189	7675	5417	4063	3160	2516	2032	1656	1355	1109	903	730	581	452	339	239	151	72
0.08	19700	9332	5876	4148	3111	2420	1926	1556	1268	1037	849	692	559	445	346	260	183	116	55
0.09	15566	7374	4643	3277	2458	1912	1522	1229	1002	820	671	547	442	352	274	205	145	92	44
0.10	12608	5973	3761	2655	1991	1549	1233	996	812	664	543	443	358	285	222	166	118	74	35
0.15	5604	2655	1672	1180	885	689	548	443	361	295	242	197	159	127	99	74	53	33	16
0.20	3152	1494	941	664	498	388	309	249	203	166	136	111	90	72	56	42	30	19	9
0.25	2018	956	602	425	319	248	198	160	130	107	87	71	58	46	36	27	19	12	6
0.30	1401	664	418	295	222	173	137	111	91	74	61	50	40	32	25	19	14	9	*
0.35	1030	488	307	217	163	127	101	82	67	55	45	37	30	24	19	14	10	7	*
0.40	788	374	236	166	125	97	78	63	51	42	34	28	23	18	14	11	8	5	*
0.50	505	239	151	107	80	62	50	40	33	27	22	18	15	12	9	7	5	*	*

* Sample size less than 5

Table 2b: Sample Size to Estimate P to Within ε Relative Percentage Points with **95%** Confidence

Anticipated Population Proportion (**P**)

ε	0.05	0.10	0.15	0.20	0.25	0.30	0.35	0.40	0.45	0.50	0.55	0.60	0.65	0.70	0.75	0.80	0.85	0.90	0.95
0.01	729904	345744	217691	153664	115249	89638	71345	57625	46953	38417	31432	25611	20686	16465	12806	9605	6780	4269	2022
0.02	182476	86436	54423	38416	28813	22410	17837	14407	11739	9605	7858	6403	5172	4117	3202	2402	1695	1068	506
0.03	81100	38416	24188	17074	12806	9960	7928	6403	5217	4269	3493	2846	2299	1830	1423	1068	754	475	225
0.04	45619	21609	13606	9604	7204	5603	4460	3602	2935	2402	1965	1601	1293	1030	801	601	424	267	127
0.05	29196	13830	8708	6147	4610	3586	2854	2305	1879	1537	1258	1025	828	659	513	385	272	171	81
0.06	20275	9604	6047	4268	3202	2490	1982	1601	1305	1068	874	712	575	458	356	267	189	119	57
0.07	14896	7056	4443	3136	2353	1830	1457	1177	959	785	642	523	423	337	262	197	139	88	42
0.08	11405	5402	3401	2401	1801	1401	1115	901	734	601	492	401	324	258	201	151	106	67	32
0.09	9011	4268	2688	1897	1423	1107	881	712	580	475	389	317	256	204	159	119	84	53	25
0.10	7299	3457	2177	1537	1153	897	714	577	470	385	315	257	207	165	129	97	68	43	21
0.15	3244	1537	968	683	513	399	318	257	209	171	140	114	92	74	57	43	31	19	9
0.20	1825	864	544	384	289	225	179	145	118	97	79	65	52	42	33	25	17	11	6
0.25	1168	553	348	246	185	144	115	93	76	62	51	41	34	27	21	16	11	7	*
0.30	811	384	242	171	129	100	80	65	53	43	35	29	23	19	15	11	8	5	*
0.35	596	282	178	125	95	74	59	48	39	32	26	21	17	14	11	8	6	*	*
0.40	456	216	136	96	73	57	45	37	30	25	20	17	13	11	9	7	5	*	*
0.50	292	138	87	61	47	36	29	24	19	16	13	11	9	7	6	*	*	*	*

* Sample size less than 5

Table 2c: Sample Size to Estimate P to Within ε Relative Percentage Points
with **90%** Confidence

Anticipated Population Proportion (**P**)

ε	0.05	0.10	0.15	0.20	0.25	0.30	0.35	0.40	0.45	0.50	0.55	0.60	0.65	0.70	0.75	0.80	0.85	0.90	0.95
0.01	514145	243543	153342	108242	81181	63141	50255	40591	33074	27061	22141	18041	14571	11598	9021	6766	4776	3007	1425
0.02	128537	60886	38336	27061	20296	15786	12564	10148	8269	6766	5536	4511	3643	2900	2256	1692	1194	752	357
0.03	57128	27061	17038	12027	9021	7016	5584	4511	3675	3007	2461	2005	1619	1289	1003	752	531	335	159
0.04	32135	15222	9584	6766	5074	3947	3141	2537	2068	1692	1384	1128	911	725	564	423	299	188	90
0.05	20566	9742	6134	4330	3248	2526	2011	1624	1323	1083	886	722	583	464	361	271	192	121	57
0.06	14282	6766	4260	3007	2256	1754	1396	1128	919	752	616	502	405	323	251	188	133	84	40
0.07	10493	4971	3130	2210	1657	1289	1026	829	675	553	452	369	298	237	185	139	98	62	30
0.08	8034	3806	2396	1692	1269	987	786	635	517	423	346	282	228	182	141	106	75	47	23
0.09	6348	3007	1894	1337	1003	780	621	502	409	335	274	223	180	144	112	84	59	38	18
0.10	5142	2436	1534	1083	812	632	503	406	331	271	222	181	146	116	91	68	48	31	15
0.15	2286	1083	682	482	361	281	224	181	147	121	99	81	65	52	41	31	22	14	7
0.20	1286	609	384	271	203	158	126	102	83	68	56	46	37	29	23	17	12	8	*
0.25	823	390	246	174	130	102	81	65	53	44	36	29	24	19	15	11	8	5	*
0.30	572	271	171	121	91	71	56	46	37	31	25	21	17	13	11	8	6	*	*
0.35	420	199	126	89	67	52	42	34	27	23	19	15	12	10	8	6	*	*	*
0.40	322	153	96	68	51	40	32	26	21	17	14	12	10	8	6	5	*	*	*
0.50	206	98	62	44	33	26	21	17	14	11	9	8	6	5	*	*	*	*	*

* Sample size less than 5

Table 3a: Sample Size for One-Sample Test of Proportion
(Level of significance: **1%**;   Power: **90%**;   Alternative hypothesis: **1-sided**)

Test Proportion (P_0)

P_a	0.05	0.10	0.15	0.20	0.25	0.30	0.35	0.40	0.45	0.50	0.55	0.60	0.65	0.70	0.75	0.80	0.85	0.90	0.95
0.10	318		591	173	87	53	36	26	20	15	12	10	8	6	5	*	*	*	*
0.15	94	535		771	215	104	62	41	29	22	17	13	10	8	6	5	*	*	*
0.20	47	147	722		925	250	117	69	45	32	23	18	13	10	8	6	5	*	*
0.25	29	70	193	883		1052	278	128	74	48	33	24	18	13	10	8	6	*	*
0.30	20	42	90	231	1018		1152	299	136	77	49	34	24	18	13	10	7	5	*
0.35	14	28	52	106	263	1126		1227	313	140	79	50	33	23	17	12	9	6	*
0.40	11	20	35	61	119	287	1208		1275	321	142	79	49	32	22	16	11	8	5
0.45	9	15	24	40	68	130	306	1264		1298	323	141	77	47	31	21	14	9	6
0.50	7	12	18	28	44	73	137	318	1294		1294	318	137	73	44	28	18	12	7
0.55	6	9	14	21	31	47	73	141	323	1298		1264	306	130	68	40	24	15	9
0.60	5	8	11	16	22	32	47	79	142	321	1275		1208	287	119	61	35	20	11
0.65	*	6	9	12	17	23	32	50	79	140	313	1227		1126	263	106	52	28	14
0.70	*	5	7	10	13	18	23	34	49	77	136	299	1152		1018	231	90	42	20
0.75	*	*	6	8	10	13	18	24	33	48	74	128	278	1052		883	193	70	29
0.80	*	*	5	6	8	10	13	18	23	32	45	69	117	250	925		722	147	47
0.85	*	*	*	5	6	8	10	13	17	22	29	41	62	104	215	771		535	94
0.90	*	*	*	*	5	6	8	10	12	15	20	26	36	53	87	173	591		318
0.95	*	*	*	*	*	5	6	7	9	11	13	17	22	29	42	66	124	382	

* Sample size less than 5

Table 3b: Sample Size for One-Sample Test of Proportion
(Level of significance: **1%**; Power: **80%**; Alternative hypothesis: **1-sided**)

Test Proportion (P_0)

P_a	0.05	0.10	0.15	0.20	0.25	0.30	0.35	0.40	0.45	0.50	0.55	0.60	0.65	0.70	0.75	0.80	0.85	0.90	0.95
0.10	231		470	140	71	44	30	22	17	13	10	8	7	5	*	*	*	*	*
0.15	66	399		607	172	83	50	34	24	18	14	11	8	7	5	*	*	*	*
0.20	32	108	546		723	197	93	55	36	25	19	14	11	8	6	5	*	*	*
0.25	19	51	143	671		819	218	101	58	38	26	19	14	11	8	6	*	*	*
0.30	13	30	66	174	777		895	233	106	60	39	26	19	14	10	7	5	*	*
0.35	10	20	38	79	199	862		951	243	109	61	39	26	18	13	9	7	*	*
0.40	7	14	25	46	90	219	927		986	249	110	61	38	25	17	12	8	5	*
0.45	6	11	18	30	51	98	234	972		1001	249	108	59	36	23	15	10	7	5
0.50	5	8	13	21	33	56	105	244	997		997	244	105	56	33	21	13	8	6
0.55	*	7	10	15	23	36	59	108	249	1001		972	234	98	51	30	18	11	7
0.60	*	5	8	12	17	25	38	61	110	249	986		927	219	90	46	25	14	10
0.65	*	*	7	9	13	18	26	39	61	109	243	951		862	199	79	38	20	13
0.70	*	*	5	7	10	14	19	26	39	60	106	233	895		777	174	66	30	13
0.75	*	*	*	6	8	11	14	19	26	38	58	101	218	819		671	143	51	19
0.80	*	*	*	5	6	8	11	14	19	25	36	55	93	197	723		546	108	32
0.85	*	*	*	*	5	7	8	11	14	18	24	34	50	83	172	607		399	66
0.90	*	*	*	*	*	5	7	8	10	13	17	22	30	44	71	140	470		231
0.95	*	*	*	*	*	*	5	6	8	9	12	15	19	25	36	56	103	311	

* Sample size less than 5

Table 3c: Sample Size for One-Sample Test of Proportion
(Level of significance: **1%**; Power: **50%**; Alternative hypothesis: **1-sided**)

Test Proportion (P_0)

P_a	0.05	0.10	0.15	0.20	0.25	0.30	0.35	0.40	0.45	0.50	0.55	0.60	0.65	0.70	0.75	0.80	0.85	0.90	0.95
0.10	103		276	87	46	29	20	15	11	9	7	6	5	*	*	*	*	*	*
0.15	26	195		347	102	51	31	21	15	12	9	7	5	*	*	*	*	*	*
0.20	12	49	276		406	114	55	33	22	16	11	9	7	5	*	*	*	*	*
0.25	7	22	69	347		455	124	58	34	22	15	11	8	6	5	*	*	*	*
0.30	5	13	31	87	406		493	130	60	34	22	15	11	8	6	*	*	*	*
0.35	*	8	18	39	102	455		520	134	61	34	21	14	10	7	5	*	*	*
0.40	*	6	12	22	46	114	493		536	136	60	33	20	13	9	6	*	*	*
0.45	*	*	8	14	26	51	124	520		542	134	58	31	19	12	8	5	*	*
0.50	*	*	6	10	17	29	55	130	536		536	130	55	29	17	10	6	*	*
0.55	*	*	5	8	12	19	31	58	134	542		520	124	51	26	14	8	*	*
0.60	*	*	*	6	9	13	20	33	60	136	536		493	114	46	22	12	6	*
0.65	*	*	*	5	7	10	14	21	34	61	134	520		455	102	39	18	8	*
0.70	*	*	*	*	6	8	11	15	22	34	60	130	493		406	87	31	13	5
0.75	*	*	*	*	5	6	8	11	15	22	34	58	124	455		347	69	22	7
0.80	*	*	*	*	*	5	7	9	11	16	22	33	55	114	406		276	49	12
0.85	*	*	*	*	*	*	5	7	9	12	15	21	31	51	102	347		195	26
0.90	*	*	*	*	*	*	5	6	7	9	11	15	20	29	46	87	276		103
0.95	*	*	*	*	*	*	*	5	6	7	9	11	14	19	26	39	69	195	103

* Sample size less than 5

Table 3d: Sample Size for One-Sample Test of Proportion

(Level of significance: **5%**; Power: **90%**; Alternative hypothesis: **1-sided**)

Test Proportion (P_0)

P_a	0.05	0.10	0.15	0.20	0.25	0.30	0.35	0.40	0.45	0.50	0.55	0.60	0.65	0.70	0.75	0.80	0.85	0.90	0.95
0.10	221		378	109	54	33	22	16	12	10	8	6	5	*	*	*	*	*	*
0.15	67	362		498	137	66	39	26	19	14	11	8	7	5	*	*	*	*	*
0.20	34	102	485		601	161	75	44	29	20	15	11	9	7	5	*	*	*	*
0.25	21	49	131	589		686	180	83	48	31	21	16	12	9	7	5	*	*	*
0.30	15	30	62	156	676		754	195	88	50	32	22	16	12	9	7	5	*	*
0.35	11	20	36	72	176	746		804	205	92	52	33	22	16	11	8	6	5	*
0.40	8	14	24	42	80	191	799		837	211	93	52	32	22	15	11	8	6	*
0.45	7	11	17	27	46	87	203	834		853	213	93	51	31	21	14	10	7	*
0.50	5	9	13	19	30	49	91	210	852		852	210	91	49	30	19	13	9	5
0.55	*	7	10	14	21	31	51	93	213	853		834	203	87	46	27	17	11	7
0.60	*	6	8	11	15	22	32	52	93	211	852		799	191	80	42	24	14	8
0.65	*	5	6	8	11	16	22	33	52	92	205	804		746	176	72	36	20	11
0.70	*	*	5	7	9	12	16	22	32	50	88	195	754		676	156	62	30	15
0.75	*	*	*	5	7	9	12	16	21	31	48	83	180	686		589	131	49	21
0.80	*	*	*	*	5	7	9	11	15	20	29	44	75	161	601		485	102	34
0.85	*	*	*	*	*	5	7	8	11	14	19	26	39	66	137	498		362	67
0.90	*	*	*	*	*	*	5	6	8	10	12	16	22	33	54	109	378		221
0.95	*	*	*	*	*	*	*	*	5	6	8	10	13	18	25	40	76	239	

* Sample size less than 5

Table 3e: Sample Size for One-Sample Test of Proportion

(Level of significance: **5%**; Power: **80%**; Alternative hypothesis: **1-sided**)

Test Proportion (P_0)

P_a	0.05	0.10	0.15	0.20	0.25	0.30	0.35	0.40	0.45	0.50	0.55	0.60	0.65	0.70	0.75	0.80	0.85	0.90	0.95
0.10	150		283	83	42	26	18	13	10	8	6	5	*	*	*	*	*	*	*
0.15	44	253		368	103	50	30	20	14	11	8	7	5	*	*	*	*	*	*
0.20	22	69	342		441	119	56	33	22	15	11	9	7	5	*	*	*	*	*
0.25	14	33	91	419		501	133	61	35	23	16	12	9	7	5	*	*	*	*
0.30	9	20	43	109	483		548	143	65	37	24	16	12	9	6	5	*	*	*
0.35	7	13	25	50	125	535		584	149	67	38	24	16	11	8	6	5	*	*
0.40	5	10	16	29	57	137	574		607	153	68	38	23	16	11	8	5	*	*
0.45	*	7	12	19	32	62	145	607		615	154	67	37	23	15	10	7	5	*
0.50	*	6	9	13	21	35	65	151	615		615	151	65	35	21	13	9	6	*
0.55	*	5	7	10	15	23	37	67	154	617		601	145	62	32	19	12	7	*
0.60	*	*	5	8	11	16	23	38	68	153	601		574	137	57	29	16	10	5
0.65	*	*	*	6	8	11	16	24	38	67	149	584		535	125	50	25	13	7
0.70	*	*	*	5	6	9	12	16	24	37	65	143	548		483	109	43	20	9
0.75	*	*	*	*	5	7	9	12	16	23	35	61	133	501		419	91	33	14
0.80	*	*	*	*	*	5	7	9	11	15	22	33	56	119	441		368	69	22
0.85	*	*	*	*	*	*	5	7	8	11	14	20	30	50	103	368		253	44
0.90	*	*	*	*	*	*	*	5	6	8	10	13	18	26	42	83	283		150
0.95	*	*	*	*	*	*	*	*	5	5	7	8	11	15	21	32	60	184	

* Sample size less than 5

Table 3f: Sample Size for One-Sample Test of Proportion
(Level of significance: **5%**; Power: **50%**; Alternative hypothesis: **1-sided**)

Test Proportion (P_0)

P_a	0.05	0.10	0.15	0.20	0.25	0.30	0.35	0.40	0.45	0.50	0.55	0.60	0.65	0.70	0.75	0.80	0.85	0.90	0.95
0.10	52		139	44	23	15	10	8	6	5	*	*	*	*	*	*	*	*	*
0.15	13	98		174	51	26	16	11	8	6	5	*	*	*	*	*	*	*	*
0.20	6	25	139		203	57	28	17	11	8	6	5	*	*	*	*	*	*	*
0.25	*	11	35	174		228	62	29	17	11	8	6	*	*	*	*	*	*	*
0.30	*	7	16	57	228		247	65	30	17	11	8	6	*	*	*	*	*	*
0.35	*	*	9	20	51	228		260	67	31	17	11	7	5	*	*	*	*	*
0.40	*	*	6	11	23	57	247		268	68	30	17	10	7	5	*	*	*	*
0.45	*	*	*	7	13	26	62	260		271	67	29	16	10	6	*	*	*	*
0.50	*	*	*	5	9	15	28	65	268		268	65	28	15	9	5	*	*	*
0.55	*	*	*	*	6	10	16	30	67	271		260	62	26	13	7	*	*	*
0.60	*	*	*	*	5	7	10	17	29	68	260		247	57	23	11	6	*	*
0.65	*	*	*	*	*	6	7	11	17	31	67	260		228	51	20	9	*	*
0.70	*	*	*	*	*	*	6	8	11	17	30	65	247		203	44	16	7	*
0.75	*	*	*	*	*	*	*	6	8	11	17	29	62	228		174	35	11	*
0.80	*	*	*	*	*	*	*	5	6	8	11	17	28	57	203		139	25	6
0.85	*	*	*	*	*	*	*	*	5	6	8	11	16	26	51	174		98	13
0.90	*	*	*	*	*	*	*	*	*	5	6	8	10	15	23	44	139		52
0.95	*	*	*	*	*	*	*	*	*	*	5	6	7	10	13	20	35	98	

* Sample size less than 5

Table 3g: Sample Size for One-Sample Test of Proportion
(Level of significance: **10%**; Power: **90%**; Alternative hypothesis: **1-sided**)

Test Proportion (P_0)

P_a	0.05	0.10	0.15	0.20	0.25	0.30	0.35	0.40	0.45	0.50	0.55	0.60	0.65	0.70	0.75	0.80	0.85	0.90	0.95
0.10	177		284	81	40	24	16	12	9	7	6	5	*	*	*	*	*	*	*
0.15	55	284		377	103	49	29	19	14	10	8	6	5	*	*	*	*	*	*
0.20	28	81	377		457	122	57	33	22	15	11	9	7	5	*	*	*	*	*
0.25	18	40	103	457		523	137	63	36	23	16	12	9	7	5	*	*	*	*
0.30	13	24	49	122	523		576	148	67	38	25	17	12	9	7	5	*	*	*
0.35	9	16	29	57	137	576		615	157	70	40	25	17	12	9	7	5	*	*
0.40	7	12	19	33	63	148	615		641	162	72	40	25	17	12	9	6	5	*
0.45	6	9	14	22	36	67	157	641		655	163	72	40	25	16	11	8	6	*
0.50	5	7	10	15	23	38	70	162	655		655	162	70	38	23	15	10	7	5
0.55	*	6	8	11	16	25	40	72	163	655		641	157	67	36	22	14	9	6
0.60	*	5	6	9	12	17	25	40	72	162	641		615	148	63	33	19	12	7
0.65	*	*	5	7	9	12	17	25	40	70	157	615		576	137	57	29	16	9
0.70	*	*	*	5	7	9	12	17	25	38	67	148	576		523	122	49	24	13
0.75	*	*	*	*	5	7	9	12	16	23	36	63	137	523		457	103	40	18
0.80	*	*	*	*	*	5	7	9	11	15	22	33	57	122	457		377	81	28
0.85	*	*	*	*	*	*	5	6	8	10	14	19	29	49	103	377		284	55
0.90	*	*	*	*	*	*	*	5	6	7	9	12	16	24	40	81	284		177
0.95	*	*	*	*	*	*	*	*	*	5	6	7	9	13	18	28	55	177	

* Sample size less than 5

Table 3h: Sample Size for One-Sample Test of Proportion
(Level of significance: **10%**; Power: **80%**; Alternative hypothesis: **1-sided**)

Test Proportion (P_0)

P_a	0.05	0.10	0.15	0.20	0.25	0.30	0.35	0.40	0.45	0.50	0.55	0.60	0.65	0.70	0.75	0.80	0.85	0.90	0.95
0.10	114		202	59	29	18	12	9	7	5	*	*	*	*	*	*	*	*	*
0.15	34	188		265	74	36	21	14	10	8	6	5	*	*	*	*	*	*	*
0.20	17	53	253		319	86	40	24	16	11	8	6	5	*	*	*	*	*	*
0.25	11	25	68	308		363	96	44	26	17	12	9	6	5	*	*	*	*	*
0.30	8	15	32	81	355		398	103	47	27	17	12	9	6	5	*	*	*	*
0.35	6	10	19	38	92	392		425	109	49	28	17	12	8	6	5	*	*	*
0.40	*	8	13	22	42	100	420		442	111	50	28	17	12	8	6	*	*	*
0.45	*	6	9	14	24	46	107	439		450	112	49	27	17	11	8	5	*	*
0.50	*	*	7	10	16	26	48	111	449		449	111	48	26	16	10	7	*	*
0.55	*	*	5	8	11	17	27	49	112	450		439	107	46	24	14	9	6	*
0.60	*	*	*	6	8	12	17	28	50	111	442		420	100	42	22	13	8	*
0.65	*	*	*	5	6	8	12	17	28	49	109	425		392	92	38	19	10	6
0.70	*	*	*	*	5	6	9	12	17	27	47	103	398		355	81	32	15	8
0.75	*	*	*	*	*	5	6	9	12	17	26	44	96	363		308	68	25	11
0.80	*	*	*	*	*	*	5	6	8	11	16	24	40	86	319		253	53	17
0.85	*	*	*	*	*	*	*	5	6	8	10	14	21	36	74	265		188	34
0.90	*	*	*	*	*	*	*	*	*	5	7	9	12	18	29	59	202		114
0.95	*	*	*	*	*	*	*	*	*	*	*	6	8	10	14	22	42	130	

* Sample size less than 5

Table 3i: Sample Size for One-Sample Test of Proportion
(Level of significance: **10%**; Power: **50%**; Alternative hypothesis: **1-sided**)

Test Proportion (P_0)

P_a	0.05	0.10	0.15	0.20	0.25	0.30	0.35	0.40	0.45	0.50	0.55	0.60	0.65	0.70	0.75	0.80	0.85	0.90	0.95
0.10	32		84	27	14	9	6	5	*	*	*	*	*	*	*	*	*	*	*
0.15	8	60		106	31	16	10	7	5	*	*	*	*	*	*	*	*	*	*
0.20	*	15	84		124	35	17	10	7	5	*	*	*	*	*	*	*	*	*
0.25	*	7	21	106		139	38	18	11	7	5	*	*	*	*	*	*	*	*
0.30	*	*	10	27	124		150	40	19	11	7	5	*	*	*	*	*	*	*
0.35	*	*	6	12	31	139		158	41	19	11	7	5	*	*	*	*	*	*
0.40	*	*	*	7	14	35	150		163	42	19	10	6	*	*	*	*	*	*
0.45	*	*	*	5	8	16	38	158		165	41	18	10	6	*	*	*	*	*
0.50	*	*	*	*	5	9	17	40	163		163	40	17	9	5	*	*	*	*
0.55	*	*	*	*	*	6	10	18	41	165		158	38	16	8	5	*	*	*
0.60	*	*	*	*	*	*	6	10	19	42	163		150	35	14	7	*	*	*
0.65	*	*	*	*	*	*	5	7	11	19	41	158		139	31	12	6	*	*
0.70	*	*	*	*	*	*	*	5	7	11	19	40	150		124	27	10	*	*
0.75	*	*	*	*	*	*	*	*	5	7	11	18	38	139		106	21	7	*
0.80	*	*	*	*	*	*	*	*	*	5	7	10	17	35	124		84	15	*
0.85	*	*	*	*	*	*	*	*	*	*	5	7	10	16	31	106		60	8
0.90	*	*	*	*	*	*	*	*	*	*	*	5	6	9	14	27	84		32
0.95	*	*	*	*	*	*	*	*	*	*	*	*	5	6	8	12	21	60	

* Sample size less than 5

Table 4a: Sample Size for One-Sample Test of Proportion
(Level of significance: **1%**; Power: **90%**; Alternative hypothesis: **2-sided**)

Test Proportion (P_0)

$\lvert P_a - P_0 \rvert$	0.05	0.10	0.15	0.20	0.25	0.30	0.35	0.40	0.45	0.50	0.55	0.60	0.65	0.70	0.75	0.80	0.85	0.90	0.95
0.01	7498	13781	19316	24105	28150	31450	34005	35816	36883	37206	36784	35618	33708	31054	27655	23512	18623	12989	6604
0.02	1974	3537	4910	6096	7095	7908	8535	8975	9230	9298	9180	8876	8386	7710	6848	5799	4563	3140	1522
0.03	919	1611	2217	2739	3178	3534	3807	3998	4105	4130	4072	3932	3708	3402	3013	2541	1985	1345	610
0.04	539	927	1266	1557	1801	1998	2149	2253	2310	2321	2286	2203	2074	1899	1677	1407	1091	726	297
0.05	358	606	821	1006	1160	1285	1379	1444	1479	1484	1459	1404	1320	1205	1061	886	681	443	127
0.10	104	166	218	262	299	328	349	363	369	368	359	343	319	287	248	201	144	60	104
0.15	52	79	101	120	136	147	156	161	163	161	156	147	135	120	101	77	101	79	52
0.20	32	47	59	69	77	83	88	90	90	88	85	79	72	62	49	27	59	47	32
0.25	22	31	39	45	50	53	56	57	56	55	52	48	42	35	20	45	39	31	22
0.30	16	22	27	32	35	37	38	39	38	37	34	31	26	16	35	32	27	22	16
0.35	12	17	20	23	25	27	27	27	27	25	23	20	13	27	25	23	20	17	12
0.40	9	13	16	18	19	20	20	20	19	18	16	10	20	20	19	18	16	13	9
0.45	8	10	12	14	15	15	15	15	14	13	14	15	15	15	15	14	12	10	8
0.50	6	8	10	11	12	12	12	11	10	7	10	11	12	12	12	11	10	8	6

Table 4b: Sample Size for One-Sample Test of Proportion
(Level of significance: **1%**; Power: **80%**; Alternative hypothesis: **2-sided**)

Test Proportion (P_0)

$\lvert P_a-P_0\rvert$	0.05	0.10	0.15	0.20	0.25	0.30	0.35	0.40	0.45	0.50	0.55	0.60	0.65	0.70	0.75	0.80	0.85	0.90	0.95
0.01	5798	10739	15093	18861	22046	24646	26662	28094	28941	29204	28884	27979	26489	24416	21758	18516	14689	10278	5277
0.02	1507	2738	3820	4756	5545	6188	6685	7036	7241	7299	7212	6978	6599	6073	5401	4583	3618	2507	1243
0.03	694	1239	1718	2131	2479	2762	2979	3132	3220	3243	3201	3094	2922	2685	2383	2016	1583	1084	513
0.04	403	709	977	1208	1402	1559	1680	1764	1812	1823	1798	1736	1637	1502	1330	1121	876	592	261
0.05	266	461	632	779	902	1002	1078	1131	1160	1166	1148	1108	1043	955	844	709	550	366	127
0.10	75	124	165	201	231	254	272	284	290	290	284	272	254	231	201	165	122	60	75
0.15	36	58	76	92	104	114	121	126	128	127	124	118	109	98	84	66	38	58	36
0.20	22	34	44	53	59	65	68	71	71	71	68	64	59	52	43	27	44	34	22
0.25	15	23	29	34	38	41	44	45	45	44	42	40	36	30	20	34	29	23	15
0.30	11	16	20	24	27	29	30	31	31	30	28	26	23	16	27	24	20	16	11
0.35	8	12	15	18	20	21	22	22	22	21	20	18	13	21	20	18	15	12	8
0.40	7	9	12	14	15	16	16	16	16	15	14	10	16	16	15	14	12	9	7
0.45	5	8	9	11	12	12	13	13	12	11	9	13	13	12	12	11	9	8	5
0.50	*	6	7	9	9	10	10	10	9	7	9	10	10	10	9	9	7	6	*

* Sample size less than 5

Table 4c: Sample Size for One-Sample Test of Proportion
(Level of significance: **1%**; Power: **50%**; Alternative hypothesis: **2-sided**)

Test Proportion (P_0)

$|P_a-P_0|$	0.05	0.10	0.15	0.20	0.25	0.30	0.35	0.40	0.45	0.50	0.55	0.60	0.65	0.70	0.75	0.80	0.85	0.90	0.95
0.01	3152	5973	8461	10618	12443	13936	15097	15926	16424	16590	16424	15926	15097	13936	12443	10618	8461	5973	3152
0.02	788	1494	2116	2655	3111	3484	3775	3982	4106	4148	4106	3982	3775	3484	3111	2655	2116	1494	788
0.03	351	664	941	1180	1383	1549	1678	1770	1825	1844	1825	1770	1678	1549	1383	1180	941	664	351
0.04	197	374	529	664	778	871	944	996	1027	1037	1027	996	944	871	778	664	529	374	197
0.05	127	239	339	425	498	558	604	638	657	664	657	638	604	558	498	425	339	239	127
0.10	32	60	85	107	125	140	151	160	165	166	165	160	151	140	125	107	85	60	32
0.15	15	27	38	48	56	62	68	71	73	74	73	71	68	62	56	48	38	27	15
0.20	8	15	22	27	32	35	38	40	42	42	42	40	38	35	32	27	22	15	8
0.25	6	10	14	17	20	23	25	26	27	27	27	26	25	23	20	17	14	10	6
0.30	*	7	10	12	14	16	17	18	19	19	19	18	17	16	14	12	10	7	*
0.35	*	5	7	9	11	12	13	14	14	14	14	14	13	12	11	9	7	5	*
0.40	*	*	6	7	8	9	10	10	11	11	11	10	10	9	8	7	6	*	*
0.45	*	*	5	6	7	7	8	8	9	9	9	8	8	7	7	6	5	*	*
0.50	*	*	*	5	5	6	7	7	7	7	7	7	7	6	5	5	*	*	*

* Sample size less than 5

Table 4d: Sample Size for One-Sample Test of Proportion
(Level of significance: **5%**; Power: **90%**; Alternative hypothesis: **2-sided**)

Test Proportion (P$_0$)

$|P_a-P_0|$	0.05	0.10	0.15	0.20	0.25	0.30	0.35	0.40	0.45	0.50	0.55	0.60	0.65	0.70	0.75	0.80	0.85	0.90	0.95
0.01	5353	9784	13686	17061	19911	22234	24032	25305	26052	26273	25968	25138	23783	21902	19495	16562	13104	9119	4603
0.02	1423	2524	3490	4324	5026	5597	6036	6344	6521	6565	6479	6261	5912	5431	4818	4074	3198	2190	1043
0.03	668	1155	1580	1947	2255	2504	2695	2827	2901	2916	2873	2771	2611	2393	2116	1780	1385	931	409
0.04	395	667	905	1109	1279	1417	1522	1594	1633	1639	1612	1552	1459	1334	1175	983	758	498	193
0.05	264	438	589	718	826	912	978	1022	1045	1047	1029	989	928	845	742	617	471	301	73
0.10	79	122	158	189	214	233	248	257	261	259	252	240	223	200	171	137	96	35	79
0.15	40	59	74	87	97	105	111	114	115	113	109	103	94	82	68	51	74	59	40
0.20	25	35	43	50	56	60	62	64	63	62	59	55	49	42	32	16	43	35	25
0.25	17	24	29	33	36	38	40	40	40	38	36	33	28	23	12	33	29	24	17
0.30	12	17	20	23	25	26	27	27	27	25	23	21	17	9	25	23	20	17	12
0.35	10	13	15	17	18	19	19	19	19	17	16	13	8	19	18	17	15	13	10
0.40	8	10	12	13	14	14	14	14	13	12	10	6	14	14	14	13	12	10	8
0.45	6	8	9	10	11	11	11	10	10	8	10	10	11	11	11	10	9	8	6
0.50	5	6	7	8	8	8	8	8	7	*	7	8	8	8	8	8	7	6	5

* Sample size less than 5

Table 4e: Sample Size for One-Sample Test of Proportion
(Level of significance: **5%**; Power: **80%**; Alternative hypothesis: **2-sided**)

Test Proportion (P_0)

$\lvert P_a - P_0 \rvert$	0.05	0.10	0.15	0.20	0.25	0.30	0.35	0.40	0.45	0.50	0.55	0.60	0.65	0.70	0.75	0.80	0.85	0.90	0.95
0.01	3933	7250	10172	12701	14837	16580	17930	18888	19453	19626	19406	18794	17789	16391	14601	12418	9842	6872	3507
0.02	1031	1856	2582	3209	3737	4167	4499	4732	4868	4905	4844	4685	4428	4072	3619	3067	2416	1667	815
0.03	478	844	1164	1440	1673	1861	2006	2107	2165	2179	2149	2076	1959	1798	1594	1346	1053	717	331
0.04	280	485	664	818	947	1052	1132	1188	1219	1225	1207	1164	1097	1005	888	747	580	389	164
0.05	185	316	430	528	610	676	727	761	780	783	771	742	698	638	563	471	363	239	73
0.10	53	86	114	137	157	172	184	191	195	194	190	182	169	153	133	108	79	35	53
0.15	26	41	53	63	71	78	82	85	86	85	83	78	72	64	54	42	22	41	26
0.20	16	24	31	36	41	44	46	48	48	47	45	43	39	34	27	16	31	24	16
0.25	11	16	20	24	26	28	30	30	30	29	28	26	23	19	12	24	20	16	11
0.30	8	12	14	17	18	20	20	21	20	20	19	17	14	9	18	17	14	12	8
0.35	6	9	11	12	13	14	15	15	15	14	13	11	8	14	13	12	11	9	6
0.40	5	7	8	9	10	11	11	11	11	10	9	6	11	11	10	9	8	7	5
0.45	*	6	7	7	8	8	8	8	8	7	5	8	8	8	8	7	7	6	*
0.50	*	5	5	6	6	7	7	6	6	*	6	6	7	7	6	6	5	5	*

* Sample size less than 5

Table 4f: Sample Size for One-Sample Test of Proportion
(Level of significance: **5%**; Power: **50%**; Alternative hypothesis: **2-sided**)

Test Proportion (P$_0$)

$|P_a-P_0|$	0.05	0.10	0.15	0.20	0.25	0.30	0.35	0.40	0.45	0.50	0.55	0.60	0.65	0.70	0.75	0.80	0.85	0.90	0.95
0.01	1825	3458	4899	6147	7204	8068	8740	9220	9508	9605	9508	9220	8740	8068	7204	6147	4899	3458	1825
0.02	457	865	1225	1537	1801	2017	2185	2305	2377	2402	2377	2305	2185	2017	1801	1537	1225	865	457
0.03	203	385	545	683	801	897	972	1025	1057	1068	1057	1025	972	897	801	683	545	385	203
0.04	115	217	307	385	451	505	547	577	595	601	595	577	547	505	451	385	307	217	115
0.05	73	139	196	246	289	323	350	369	381	385	381	369	350	323	289	246	196	139	73
0.10	19	35	49	62	73	81	88	93	96	97	96	93	88	81	73	62	49	35	19
0.15	9	16	22	28	33	36	39	41	43	43	43	41	39	36	33	28	22	16	9
0.20	5	9	13	16	19	21	22	24	24	25	24	24	22	21	19	16	13	9	5
0.25	*	6	8	10	12	13	14	15	16	16	16	15	14	13	12	10	8	6	*
0.30	*	*	6	7	9	9	10	11	11	11	11	11	10	9	9	7	6	*	*
0.35	*	*	*	6	6	7	8	8	8	8	8	8	8	7	6	6	*	*	*
0.40	*	*	*	*	5	6	6	6	6	7	6	6	6	6	5	*	*	*	*
0.45	*	*	*	*	*	*	5	5	5	5	5	5	5	*	5	*	*	*	*
0.50	*	*	*	*	*	*	*	*	*	*	*	*	*	*	*	*	*	*	*

* Sample size less than 5

Table 4g: Sample Size for One-Sample Test of Proportion

(Level of significance: **10%**; Power: **90%**; Alternative hypothesis: **2-sided**)

Test Proportion (P_0)

$|P_a-P_0|$	0.05	0.10	0.15	0.20	0.25	0.30	0.35	0.40	0.45	0.50	0.55	0.60	0.65	0.70	0.75	0.80	0.85	0.90	0.95
0.01	4396	8004	11181	13928	16247	18138	19600	20633	21238	21415	21163	20483	19375	17838	15872	13478	10655	7403	3718
0.02	1176	2071	2857	3535	4106	4569	4926	5175	5317	5351	5279	5100	4813	4419	3918	3310	2594	1770	833
0.03	555	950	1296	1594	1844	2045	2200	2306	2365	2377	2340	2256	2125	1945	1718	1443	1120	749	322
0.04	329	551	743	909	1047	1158	1243	1301	1331	1335	1313	1263	1186	1083	953	796	611	398	148
0.05	221	362	485	589	676	746	799	834	852	853	837	804	754	686	601	498	378	239	52
0.10	67	102	131	156	176	191	203	210	213	211	205	195	180	161	137	109	76	25	67
0.15	34	49	62	72	80	87	91	93	93	92	88	83	75	66	54	40	62	49	34
0.20	21	30	36	42	46	49	51	52	52	50	48	44	39	33	25	11	36	30	21
0.25	15	20	24	27	30	31	32	33	32	31	29	26	22	18	9	27	24	20	15
0.30	11	14	17	19	21	22	22	22	21	20	19	16	13	7	21	19	17	14	11
0.35	8	11	13	14	15	16	16	16	15	14	12	10	6	16	15	14	13	11	8
0.40	7	9	10	11	11	12	12	11	11	10	8	5	12	12	11	11	10	9	7
0.45	5	7	8	8	9	9	9	8	8	6	8	8	9	9	9	8	8	7	5
0.50	*	6	6	7	7	7	7	6	5	*	5	6	7	7	7	7	6	6	*

* Sample size less than 5

Table 4h: Sample Size for One-Sample Test of Proportion
(Level of significance: **10%**; Power: **80%**; Alternative hypothesis: **2-sided**)

Test Proportion (P_0)

$|P_a-P_0|$	0.05	0.10	0.15	0.20	0.25	0.30	0.35	0.40	0.45	0.50	0.55	0.60	0.65	0.70	0.75	0.80	0.85	0.90	0.95
0.01	3120	5730	8030	10020	11700	13071	14132	14885	15328	15461	15286	14801	14007	12903	11490	9768	7737	5395	2741
0.02	822	1472	2042	2535	2950	3287	3548	3730	3836	3864	3815	3688	3485	3203	2845	2409	1895	1303	631
0.03	383	671	922	1139	1321	1469	1583	1662	1706	1717	1692	1634	1541	1413	1252	1055	824	558	253
0.04	225	386	527	648	749	831	893	937	960	965	950	916	862	789	696	585	453	301	123
0.05	150	253	342	419	483	535	574	601	615	617	607	584	548	501	441	368	283	184	52
0.10	44	69	91	109	125	137	145	151	154	153	149	143	133	119	103	83	60	25	44
0.15	22	33	43	50	57	62	65	67	68	67	65	61	56	50	42	32	16	33	22
0.20	14	20	25	29	32	35	37	38	38	37	35	33	30	26	21	11	25	20	14
0.25	9	13	16	19	21	23	23	24	24	23	22	20	18	15	9	19	16	13	9
0.30	7	10	12	13	15	16	16	16	16	15	14	13	11	7	15	13	12	10	7
0.35	5	7	9	10	11	11	12	12	11	11	10	8	6	11	11	10	9	7	5
0.40	*	6	7	8	8	9	9	9	8	8	7	5	9	9	8	8	7	6	*
0.45	*	5	5	6	6	7	7	7	6	5	6	7	7	7	6	6	5	5	*
0.50	*	*	*	5	5	5	5	5	5	*	5	5	5	5	5	5	*	*	*

* Sample size less than 5

Table 4i: Sample Size for One-Sample Test of Proportion
(Level of significance: **10%**; Power: **50%**; Alternative hypothesis: **2-sided**)

Test Proportion (P_0)

$|P_a-P_0|$	0.05	0.10	0.15	0.20	0.25	0.30	0.35	0.40	0.45	0.50	0.55	0.60	0.65	0.70	0.75	0.80	0.85	0.90	0.95
0.01	1286	2436	3451	4330	5074	5683	6157	6495	6698	6766	6698	6495	6157	5683	5074	4330	3451	2436	1286
0.02	322	609	863	1083	1269	1421	1540	1624	1675	1692	1675	1624	1540	1421	1269	1083	863	609	322
0.03	143	271	384	482	564	632	685	722	745	752	745	722	685	632	564	482	384	271	143
0.04	81	153	216	271	318	356	385	406	419	423	419	406	385	356	318	271	216	153	81
0.05	52	98	139	174	203	228	247	260	268	271	268	260	247	228	203	174	139	98	52
0.10	13	25	35	44	51	57	62	65	67	68	67	65	62	57	51	44	35	25	13
0.15	6	11	16	20	23	26	28	29	30	31	30	29	28	26	23	20	16	11	6
0.20	*	7	9	11	13	15	16	17	17	17	17	17	16	15	13	11	9	7	*
0.25	*	*	6	7	9	10	10	11	11	11	11	11	10	10	9	7	6	*	*
0.30	*	*	*	5	6	7	7	8	8	8	8	8	7	7	6	5	*	*	*
0.35	*	*	*	*	5	5	6	6	6	6	6	6	6	5	5	*	*	*	*
0.40	*	*	*	*	*	*	*	5	5	5	5	5	*	*	*	*	*	*	*
0.45	*	*	*	*	*	*	*	*	*	*	*	*	*	*	*	*	*	*	*
0.50	*	*	*	*	*	*	*	*	*	*	*	*	*	*	*	*	*	*	*

* Sample size less than 5

Table 5a: Values of V [V = $P_1(1-P_1) + P_2(1-P_2)$]

P$_2$ or (1-P$_2$)

P$_1$ or (1-P$_1$)	0.01	0.02	0.03	0.04	0.05	0.10	0.15	0.20	0.25	0.30	0.35	0.40	0.45	0.50
0.01	0.02	0.03	0.04	0.05	0.06	0.10	0.14	0.17	0.20	0.22	0.24	0.25	0.26	0.26
0.02	0.03	0.04	0.05	0.06	0.07	0.11	0.15	0.18	0.21	0.23	0.25	0.26	0.27	0.27
0.03	0.04	0.05	0.06	0.07	0.08	0.12	0.16	0.19	0.22	0.24	0.26	0.27	0.28	0.28
0.04	0.05	0.06	0.07	0.08	0.09	0.13	0.17	0.20	0.23	0.25	0.27	0.28	0.29	0.29
0.05	0.06	0.07	0.08	0.09	0.10	0.14	0.18	0.21	0.24	0.26	0.28	0.29	0.30	0.30
0.06	0.07	0.08	0.09	0.09	0.10	0.15	0.18	0.22	0.24	0.27	0.28	0.30	0.30	0.31
0.07	0.08	0.08	0.09	0.10	0.11	0.16	0.19	0.23	0.25	0.28	0.29	0.31	0.31	0.32
0.08	0.08	0.09	0.10	0.11	0.12	0.16	0.20	0.23	0.26	0.28	0.30	0.31	0.32	0.32
0.09	0.09	0.10	0.11	0.12	0.13	0.17	0.21	0.24	0.27	0.29	0.31	0.32	0.33	0.33
0.10	0.10	0.11	0.12	0.13	0.14	0.18	0.22	0.25	0.28	0.30	0.32	0.33	0.34	0.34
0.12	0.12	0.13	0.13	0.14	0.15	0.20	0.23	0.27	0.29	0.32	0.33	0.35	0.35	0.36
0.14	0.13	0.14	0.15	0.16	0.17	0.21	0.25	0.28	0.31	0.33	0.35	0.36	0.37	0.37
0.16	0.14	0.15	0.16	0.17	0.18	0.22	0.26	0.29	0.32	0.34	0.36	0.37	0.38	0.38
0.18	0.16	0.17	0.18	0.19	0.20	0.24	0.28	0.31	0.34	0.36	0.38	0.39	0.40	0.40
0.20	0.17	0.18	0.19	0.20	0.21	0.25	0.29	0.32	0.35	0.37	0.39	0.40	0.41	0.41
0.22	0.18	0.19	0.20	0.21	0.22	0.26	0.30	0.33	0.36	0.38	0.40	0.41	0.42	0.42
0.24	0.19	0.20	0.21	0.22	0.23	0.27	0.31	0.34	0.37	0.39	0.41	0.42	0.43	0.43
0.26	0.20	0.21	0.22	0.23	0.24	0.28	0.32	0.35	0.38	0.40	0.42	0.43	0.44	0.44
0.28	0.21	0.22	0.23	0.24	0.25	0.29	0.33	0.36	0.39	0.41	0.43	0.44	0.45	0.45
0.30	0.22	0.23	0.24	0.25	0.26	0.30	0.34	0.37	0.40	0.42	0.44	0.45	0.46	0.46
0.32	0.23	0.24	0.25	0.26	0.27	0.31	0.35	0.38	0.41	0.43	0.45	0.46	0.47	0.47
0.34	0.23	0.24	0.25	0.26	0.27	0.31	0.35	0.38	0.41	0.43	0.45	0.46	0.47	0.47
0.36	0.24	0.25	0.26	0.27	0.28	0.32	0.36	0.39	0.42	0.44	0.46	0.47	0.48	0.48
0.38	0.25	0.26	0.26	0.27	0.28	0.33	0.36	0.40	0.42	0.45	0.46	0.48	0.48	0.49
0.40	0.25	0.26	0.27	0.28	0.29	0.33	0.37	0.40	0.43	0.45	0.47	0.48	0.49	0.49
0.42	0.25	0.26	0.27	0.28	0.29	0.33	0.37	0.40	0.43	0.45	0.47	0.48	0.49	0.49
0.44	0.26	0.27	0.28	0.28	0.29	0.34	0.37	0.41	0.43	0.46	0.47	0.49	0.49	0.50
0.46	0.26	0.27	0.28	0.29	0.30	0.34	0.38	0.41	0.44	0.46	0.48	0.49	0.50	0.50
0.48	0.26	0.27	0.28	0.29	0.30	0.34	0.38	0.41	0.44	0.46	0.48	0.49	0.50	0.50
0.50	0.26	0.27	0.28	0.29	0.30	0.34	0.38	0.41	0.44	0.46	0.48	0.49	0.50	0.50

Table 5b: Sample Size to Estimate the Risk Difference Between Two Proportions, P_1 and P_2, to Within **d** Percentage Points with **99%** Confidence [Using $V = P_1(1-P_1) + P_2(1-P_2)$]

V	\multicolumn{14}{c}{d%}
	1	2	3	4	5	10	15	20	25	30	35	40	45	50
0.01	664	166	74	42	27	7	*	*	*	*	*	*	*	*
0.02	1328	332	148	83	54	14	6	*	*	*	*	*	*	*
0.03	1991	498	222	125	80	20	9	5	*	*	*	*	*	*
0.04	2655	664	295	166	107	27	12	7	5	*	*	*	*	*
0.05	3318	830	369	208	133	34	15	9	6	*	*	*	*	*
0.06	3982	996	443	249	160	40	18	10	7	5	*	*	*	*
0.07	4646	1162	517	291	186	47	21	12	8	6	*	*	*	*
0.08	5309	1328	590	332	213	54	24	14	9	6	5	*	*	*
0.09	5973	1494	664	374	239	60	27	15	10	7	5	*	*	*
0.10	6636	1659	738	415	266	67	30	17	11	8	6	5	*	*
0.12	7963	1991	885	498	319	80	36	20	13	9	7	5	*	*
0.14	9291	2323	1033	581	372	93	42	24	15	11	8	6	5	*
0.16	10618	2655	1180	664	425	107	48	27	17	12	9	7	6	5
0.18	11945	2987	1328	747	478	120	54	30	20	14	10	8	6	5
0.20	13272	3318	1475	830	531	133	59	34	22	15	11	9	7	6
0.22	14599	3650	1623	913	584	146	65	37	24	17	12	10	8	6
0.24	15926	3982	1770	996	638	160	71	40	26	18	14	10	8	7
0.26	17254	4314	1918	1079	691	173	77	44	28	20	15	11	9	7
0.28	18581	4646	2065	1162	744	186	83	47	30	21	16	12	10	8
0.30	19908	4977	2212	1245	797	200	89	50	32	23	17	13	10	8
0.32	21235	5309	2360	1328	850	213	95	54	34	24	18	14	11	9
0.34	22562	5641	2507	1411	903	226	101	57	37	26	19	15	12	10
0.36	23889	5973	2655	1494	956	239	107	60	39	27	20	15	12	10
0.38	25216	6304	2802	1576	1009	253	113	64	41	29	21	16	13	11
0.40	26544	6636	2950	1659	1062	266	118	67	43	30	22	17	14	11
0.42	27871	6968	3097	1742	1115	279	124	70	45	31	23	18	14	12
0.44	29198	7300	3245	1825	1168	292	130	73	47	33	24	19	15	12
0.46	30525	7632	3392	1908	1221	306	136	77	49	34	25	20	16	13
0.48	31852	7963	3540	1991	1275	319	142	80	51	36	27	20	16	13
0.50	33179	8295	3687	2074	1328	332	148	83	54	37	28	21	17	14

*Sample size less than 5

Table 5c: Sample Size to Estimate the Risk Difference Between Two Proportions, P_1 and P_2, to Within **d** Percentage Points with **95%** Confidence [Using $V = P_1(1-P_1) + P_2(1-P_2)$]

V	\multicolumn{14}{c}{d%}													
	1	2	3	4	5	10	15	20	25	30	35	40	45	50
0.01	385	97	43	25	16	*	*	*	*	*	*	*	*	*
0.02	769	193	86	49	31	8	*	*	*	*	*	*	*	*
0.03	1153	289	129	73	47	12	6	*	*	*	*	*	*	*
0.04	1537	385	171	97	62	16	7	*	*	*	*	*	*	*
0.05	1921	481	214	121	77	20	9	5	*	*	*	*	*	*
0.06	2305	577	257	145	93	24	11	6	*	*	*	*	*	*
0.07	2690	673	299	169	108	27	12	7	5	*	*	*	*	*
0.08	3074	769	342	193	123	31	14	8	5	*	*	*	*	*
0.09	3458	865	385	217	139	35	16	9	6	5	*	*	*	*
0.10	3842	961	427	241	154	39	18	10	7	6	*	*	*	*
0.12	4610	1153	513	289	185	47	21	12	8	6	5	*	*	*
0.14	5379	1345	598	337	216	54	24	14	9	7	6	*	*	*
0.16	6147	1537	683	385	246	62	28	16	10	8	6	5	*	*
0.18	6915	1729	769	433	277	70	31	18	12	8	7	5	*	*
0.20	7684	1921	854	481	308	77	35	20	13	9	7	5	5	*
0.22	8452	2113	940	529	339	85	38	22	14	10	8	6	5	*
0.24	9220	2305	1025	577	369	93	41	24	15	11	9	6	5	*
0.26	9989	2498	1110	625	400	100	45	25	16	12	9	6	5	5
0.28	10757	2690	1196	673	431	108	48	27	18	12	10	7	6	5
0.30	11525	2882	1281	721	461	116	52	29	19	13	10	7	6	5
0.32	12294	3074	1366	769	492	123	55	31	20	14	11	8	6	6
0.34	13062	3266	1452	817	523	131	59	33	21	15	11	8	7	6
0.36	13830	3458	1537	865	554	139	62	35	23	16	12	9	7	6
0.38	14599	3650	1623	913	584	146	65	37	24	17	12	9	7	6
0.40	15367	3842	1708	961	615	154	69	39	25	18	13	10	8	7
0.42	16135	4034	1793	1009	646	162	72	41	26	18	14	10	8	7
0.44	16904	4226	1879	1057	677	170	76	43	28	19	14	11	8	7
0.46	17672	4418	1964	1105	707	177	79	45	29	20	15	11	9	8
0.48	18440	4610	2049	1153	738	185	82	47	30	21	16	12	10	8
0.50	19209	4803	2135	1201	769	193	86	49	31	22	16	13	10	8

Table 5d: Sample Size to Estimate the Risk Difference Between Two Proportions, P_1 and P_2, to Within **d** Percentage Points with **90%** Confidence [Using $V = P_1(1-P_1) + P_2(1-P_2)$]

d%

V	1	2	3	4	5	10	15	20	25	30	35	40	45	50
0.01	271	68	31	17	11	*	*	*	*	*	*	*	*	*
0.02	542	136	61	34	22	6	*	*	*	*	*	*	*	*
0.03	812	203	91	51	33	9	*	*	*	*	*	*	*	*
0.04	1083	271	121	68	44	11	5	*	*	*	*	*	*	*
0.05	1354	339	151	85	55	14	7	*	*	*	*	*	*	*
0.06	1624	406	181	102	65	17	8	5	*	*	*	*	*	*
0.07	1895	474	211	119	76	19	9	5	*	*	*	*	*	*
0.08	2165	542	241	136	87	22	10	6	*	*	*	*	*	*
0.09	2436	609	271	153	98	25	11	7	*	*	*	*	*	*
0.10	2707	677	301	170	109	28	13	7	5	*	*	*	*	*
0.12	3248	812	361	203	130	33	15	9	6	*	*	*	*	*
0.14	3789	948	421	237	152	38	17	10	7	5	*	*	*	*
0.16	4330	1083	482	271	174	44	20	11	7	5	*	*	*	*
0.18	4871	1218	542	305	195	49	22	13	8	6	*	*	*	*
0.20	5413	1354	602	339	217	55	25	14	9	7	5	*	*	*
0.22	5954	1489	662	373	239	60	27	15	10	7	5	*	*	*
0.24	6495	1624	722	406	260	65	29	17	11	8	6	5	*	*
0.26	7036	1759	782	440	282	71	32	18	12	8	6	5	*	*
0.28	7577	1895	842	474	304	76	34	19	13	9	7	5	*	*
0.30	8119	2030	903	508	325	82	37	21	13	10	7	6	5	*
0.32	8660	2165	963	542	347	87	39	22	14	10	8	6	5	*
0.34	9201	2301	1023	576	369	93	41	24	15	11	8	6	5	*
0.36	9742	2436	1083	609	390	98	44	25	16	11	8	7	5	*
0.38	10283	2571	1143	643	412	103	46	26	17	12	9	7	6	5
0.40	10825	2707	1203	677	433	109	49	28	18	13	9	7	6	5
0.42	11366	2842	1263	711	455	114	51	29	19	13	10	8	6	5
0.44	11907	2977	1323	745	477	120	53	30	20	14	10	8	6	5
0.46	12448	3112	1384	778	498	125	56	32	20	14	11	8	7	5
0.48	12989	3248	1444	812	520	130	58	33	21	15	11	9	7	6
0.50	13531	3383	1504	846	542	136	61	34	22	16	12	9	7	6

*Sample size less than 5

Table 6a: Sample Size for Two-Sample Test of Proportions
(Level of significance: **1%**; Power: **90%**; Alternative hypothesis: **1-sided**)

P_1

P_2	0.05	0.10	0.15	0.20	0.25	0.30	0.35	0.40	0.45	0.50	0.55	0.60	0.65	0.70	0.75	0.80	0.85	0.90	0.95
0.10	721		1137	330	165	102	71	52	40	32	26	22	18	15	13	11	9	8	7
0.15	232	1137		1502	415	200	120	81	59	45	35	28	23	19	16	13	11	9	8
0.20	125	330	1502		1814	486	229	135	90	64	48	37	30	24	20	16	13	11	9
0.25	81	165	415	1814		2075	545	252	146	96	68	50	38	30	24	20	16	13	11
0.30	58	102	200	486	2075		2283	590	269	154	100	70	51	39	30	24	19	15	12
0.35	44	71	120	229	545	2283		2439	623	281	159	102	70	51	38	30	23	18	14
0.40	35	52	81	135	252	590	2439		2543	643	287	161	102	70	50	37	28	22	17
0.45	29	40	59	90	146	269	623	2543		2595	649	287	159	100	68	48	35	26	20
0.50	24	32	45	64	96	154	281	643	2595		2595	643	281	154	96	64	45	32	24
0.55	20	26	35	48	68	100	159	287	649	2595		2543	623	269	146	90	59	40	29
0.60	17	22	28	37	50	70	102	161	287	643	2543		2439	590	252	135	81	52	35
0.65	14	18	23	30	38	51	70	102	159	281	623	2439		2283	545	229	120	71	44
0.70	12	15	19	24	30	39	51	70	100	154	269	590	2283		2075	486	200	102	58
0.75	11	13	16	20	24	30	38	50	68	96	146	252	545	2075		1814	415	165	81
0.80	9	11	13	16	20	24	30	37	48	64	90	135	229	486	1814		1502	330	125
0.85	8	9	11	13	16	19	23	28	35	45	59	81	120	200	415	1502		1137	232
0.90	7	8	9	11	13	15	18	22	26	32	40	52	71	102	165	330	1137		721
0.95	6	7	8	9	11	12	14	17	20	24	29	35	44	58	81	125	232	721	

Table 6b: Sample Size for Two-Sample Test of Proportions
(Level of significance: **1%**; Power: **80%**; Alternative hypothesis: **1-sided**)

P_1

P_2	0.05	0.10	0.15	0.20	0.25	0.30	0.35	0.40	0.45	0.50	0.55	0.60	0.65	0.70	0.75	0.80	0.85	0.90	0.95
0.10	556		877	255	128	79	55	41	32	25	21	17	15	12	11	9	8	7	6
0.15	180	877		1158	320	155	93	63	46	35	28	22	18	15	13	11	9	8	7
0.20	97	255	1158		1399	376	177	105	70	50	38	29	23	19	16	13	11	9	8
0.25	63	128	320	1399		1600	421	195	113	74	53	39	30	24	19	16	13	11	9
0.30	46	79	155	376	1600		1761	456	208	120	78	54	40	30	24	19	15	12	10
0.35	35	55	93	177	421	1761		1881	481	217	123	79	55	40	30	23	18	15	12
0.40	28	41	63	105	195	456	1881		1961	496	222	125	79	54	39	29	22	17	14
0.45	23	32	46	70	113	208	481	1961		2001	501	222	123	78	53	38	28	21	16
0.50	19	25	35	50	74	120	217	496	2001		2001	496	217	120	74	50	35	25	19
0.55	16	21	28	38	53	78	123	222	501	2001		1961	481	208	113	70	46	32	23
0.60	14	17	22	29	39	54	79	125	222	496	1961		1881	456	195	105	63	41	28
0.65	12	15	18	23	30	40	55	79	123	217	481	1881		1761	421	177	93	55	35
0.70	10	12	15	19	24	30	40	54	78	120	208	456	1761		1600	376	155	79	46
0.75	9	11	13	16	19	24	30	39	53	74	113	195	421	1600		1399	320	128	63
0.80	8	9	11	13	16	19	23	29	38	50	70	105	177	376	1399		1158	255	97
0.85	7	8	9	11	13	15	18	22	28	35	46	63	93	155	320	1158		877	180
0.90	6	7	8	9	11	12	15	17	21	25	32	41	55	79	128	255	877		556
0.95	5	6	7	8	9	10	12	14	16	19	23	28	35	46	63	97	180	556	

Table 6c: Sample Size for Two-Sample Test of Proportions
(Level of significance: **1%**; Power: **50%**; Alternative hypothesis: **1-sided**)

P_1

P_2	0.05	0.10	0.15	0.20	0.25	0.30	0.35	0.40	0.45	0.50	0.55	0.60	0.65	0.70	0.75	0.80	0.85	0.90	0.95
0.10	301		474	138	70	44	31	23	18	15	12	10	9	8	7	6	5	5	*
0.15	98	474		625	174	84	51	35	26	20	16	13	11	9	8	7	6	5	5
0.20	53	138	625		755	203	96	57	38	28	21	17	14	11	9	8	7	6	5
0.25	35	70	174	755		863	228	106	62	41	29	22	17	14	11	9	8	7	6
0.30	25	44	84	203	863		950	247	113	65	43	30	23	17	14	11	9	8	7
0.35	20	31	51	96	228	950		1015	260	118	67	44	31	23	17	14	11	9	7
0.40	16	23	35	57	106	247	1015		1058	268	120	68	44	30	22	17	13	10	8
0.45	13	18	26	38	62	113	260	1058		1080	271	120	67	43	29	21	16	12	10
0.50	11	15	20	28	41	65	118	268	1080		1080	268	118	65	41	28	20	15	11
0.55	10	12	16	21	29	43	67	120	271	1080		1058	260	113	62	38	26	18	13
0.60	8	10	13	17	22	30	44	68	120	268	1058		1015	247	106	57	35	23	16
0.65	7	9	11	14	17	23	31	44	67	118	260	1015		950	228	96	51	31	20
0.70	7	8	9	11	14	17	23	30	43	65	113	247	950		863	203	84	44	25
0.75	6	7	8	9	11	14	17	22	29	41	62	106	228	863		755	174	70	35
0.80	5	6	7	8	9	11	14	17	21	28	38	57	96	203	755		625	138	53
0.85	5	5	6	7	8	9	11	13	16	20	26	35	51	84	174	625		474	98
0.90	*	5	5	6	7	8	9	10	12	15	18	23	31	44	70	138	474		301
0.95	*	*	5	5	6	7	7	8	10	11	13	16	20	25	35	53	98	301	

* Sample size less than 5

Table 6d: Sample Size for Two-Sample Test of Proportions
(Level of significance: **5%**; Power: **90%**; Alternative hypothesis: **1-sided**)

P_1

P_2	0.05	0.10	0.15	0.20	0.25	0.30	0.35	0.40	0.45	0.50	0.55	0.60	0.65	0.70	0.75	0.80	0.85	0.90	0.95
0.10	474		748	217	109	67	46	34	26	21	17	14	12	10	8	7	6	5	*
0.15	153	748		988	273	131	79	53	39	29	23	18	15	12	10	9	7	6	5
0.20	82	217	988		1194	320	150	89	59	42	31	24	19	16	13	10	9	7	6
0.25	53	109	273	1194		1365	358	166	96	63	44	33	25	20	16	13	10	8	7
0.30	38	67	131	320	1365		1502	388	177	101	66	46	33	25	20	16	12	10	8
0.35	29	46	79	150	358	1502		1605	410	185	105	67	46	33	25	19	15	12	9
0.40	23	34	53	89	166	388	1605		1674	423	189	106	67	46	33	24	18	14	11
0.45	19	26	39	59	96	177	410	1674		1708	427	189	105	66	44	31	23	17	13
0.50	15	21	29	42	63	101	185	423	1708		1708	423	185	101	63	42	29	21	15
0.55	13	17	23	31	44	66	105	189	427	1708		1674	410	177	96	59	39	26	19
0.60	11	14	18	24	33	46	67	106	189	423	1674		1605	388	166	89	53	34	23
0.65	9	12	15	19	25	33	46	67	105	185	410	1605		1502	358	150	79	46	29
0.70	8	10	12	16	20	25	33	46	66	101	177	388	1502		1365	320	131	67	38
0.75	7	8	10	13	16	20	25	33	44	63	96	166	358	1365		1194	273	109	53
0.80	6	7	9	10	13	16	19	24	31	42	59	89	150	320	1194		988	217	82
0.85	5	6	7	9	10	12	15	18	23	29	39	53	79	131	273	988		748	153
0.90	*	5	6	7	8	10	12	14	17	21	26	34	46	67	109	217	748		474
0.95	*	*	5	6	7	8	9	11	13	15	19	23	29	38	53	82	153	474	

* Sample size less than 5

Table 6e: Sample Size for Two-Sample Test of Proportions
(Level of significance: **5%**; Power: **80%**; Alternative hypothesis: **1-sided**)

P_1

P_2	0.05	0.10	0.15	0.20	0.25	0.30	0.35	0.40	0.45	0.50	0.55	0.60	0.65	0.70	0.75	0.80	0.85	0.90	0.95
0.10	343		541	157	79	49	34	25	20	16	13	11	9	8	7	6	5	*	*
0.15	111	541		714	197	95	57	39	28	22	17	14	11	9	8	7	6	5	*
0.20	60	157	714		862	231	109	64	43	31	23	18	14	12	10	8	7	6	5
0.25	39	79	197	862		986	259	120	70	46	32	24	19	15	12	10	8	7	5
0.30	28	49	95	231	986		1085	281	128	74	48	33	25	19	15	12	9	8	6
0.35	21	34	57	109	259	1085		1159	296	134	76	49	34	25	19	14	11	9	7
0.40	17	25	39	64	120	281	1159		1209	306	137	77	49	33	24	18	14	11	8
0.45	14	20	28	43	70	128	296	1209		1233	309	137	76	48	32	23	17	13	10
0.50	12	16	22	31	46	74	134	306	1233		1233	306	134	74	46	31	22	16	12
0.55	10	13	17	23	32	48	76	137	309	1233		1209	296	128	70	43	28	20	14
0.60	8	11	14	18	24	33	49	77	137	306	1209		1159	281	120	64	39	25	17
0.65	7	9	11	14	19	25	34	49	76	134	296	1159		1085	259	109	57	34	21
0.70	6	8	9	12	15	19	25	33	48	74	128	281	1085		986	231	95	49	28
0.75	5	7	8	10	12	15	19	24	32	46	70	120	259	986		862	197	79	39
0.80	5	6	7	8	10	12	14	18	23	31	43	64	109	231	862		714	157	60
0.85	*	5	6	7	8	9	11	14	17	22	28	39	57	95	197	714		541	111
0.90	*	*	5	6	7	8	9	11	13	16	20	25	34	49	79	157	541		343
0.95	*	*	*	5	5	6	7	8	10	12	14	17	21	28	39	60	111	343	

* Sample size less than 5

Table 6f: Sample Size for Two-Sample Test of Proportions
(Level of significance: **5%**; Power: **50%**; Alternative hypothesis: **1-sided**)

P_1

P_2	0.05	0.10	0.15	0.20	0.25	0.30	0.35	0.40	0.45	0.50	0.55	0.60	0.65	0.70	0.75	0.80	0.85	0.90	0.95
0.10	151		237	70	35	22	16	12	9	8	6	5	5	*	*	*	*	*	*
0.15	49	237		313	87	42	26	18	13	10	8	7	6	5	*	*	*	*	*
0.20	27	70	313		378	102	48	29	19	14	11	9	7	6	5	*	*	*	*
0.25	18	35	87	378		432	114	53	31	21	15	11	9	7	6	5	*	*	*
0.30	13	22	42	102	432		475	124	57	33	22	15	12	9	7	6	5	*	*
0.35	10	16	26	48	114	475		508	130	59	34	22	16	12	9	7	6	5	*
0.40	8	12	18	29	53	124	508		530	134	60	34	22	15	11	9	7	5	5
0.45	7	9	13	19	31	57	130	530		540	136	60	34	22	15	11	8	6	5
0.50	6	8	10	14	21	33	59	134	540		540	134	59	33	21	14	10	8	6
0.55	5	6	8	11	15	22	34	60	136	540		530	130	57	31	19	13	9	7
0.60	*	5	7	9	11	15	22	34	60	134	530		508	124	53	29	18	12	8
0.65	*	5	6	7	9	12	16	22	34	59	130	508		475	114	48	26	16	10
0.70	*	*	5	6	7	9	12	15	22	33	57	124	475		432	102	42	22	13
0.75	*	*	*	5	6	7	9	11	15	21	31	53	114	432		378	87	35	18
0.80	*	*	*	*	5	6	7	9	11	14	19	29	48	102	378		313	70	27
0.85	*	*	*	*	*	5	6	7	8	10	13	18	26	42	87	313		237	49
0.90	*	*	*	*	*	*	5	5	6	8	9	12	16	22	35	70	237		151
0.95	*	*	*	*	*	*	*	5	5	6	7	8	10	13	18	27	49	151	

* Sample size less than 5

Table 6g: Sample Size for Two-Sample Test of Proportions
(Level of significance:**10%**; Power: **90%**; Alternative hypothesis: **1-sided**)

P_2	\multicolumn{19}{c}{P_1}

P_2	0.05	0.10	0.15	0.20	0.25	0.30	0.35	0.40	0.45	0.50	0.55	0.60	0.65	0.70	0.75	0.80	0.85	0.90	0.95
0.10	364		574	166	83	51	36	26	20	16	13	11	9	8	7	5	5	*	*
0.15	117	574		758	209	101	60	41	30	22	18	14	11	9	8	7	5	5	*
0.20	63	166	758		916	245	115	68	45	32	24	19	15	12	10	8	7	5	*
0.25	41	83	209	916		1047	275	127	74	48	34	25	19	15	12	10	8	6	5
0.30	29	51	101	245	1047		1153	298	136	78	50	35	26	19	15	12	9	8	6
0.35	22	36	60	115	275	1153		1231	314	142	80	51	35	26	19	15	11	9	7
0.40	18	26	41	68	127	298	1231		1284	324	145	81	51	35	25	19	14	11	8
0.45	14	20	30	45	74	136	314	1284		1310	328	145	80	50	34	24	18	13	10
0.50	12	16	22	32	48	78	142	324	1310		1310	324	142	78	48	32	22	16	12
0.55	10	13	18	24	34	50	80	145	328	1310		1284	314	136	74	45	30	20	14
0.60	8	11	14	19	25	35	51	81	145	324	1284		1231	298	127	68	41	26	18
0.65	7	9	11	15	19	26	35	51	80	142	314	1231		1153	275	115	60	36	22
0.70	6	8	9	12	15	19	26	35	50	78	136	298	1153		1047	245	101	51	29
0.75	5	7	8	10	12	15	19	25	34	48	74	127	275	1047		916	209	83	41
0.80	*	5	7	8	10	12	15	19	24	32	45	68	115	245	916		758	166	63
0.85	*	5	5	7	8	9	11	14	18	22	30	41	60	101	209	758		574	117
0.90	*	*	5	5	6	8	9	11	13	16	20	26	36	51	83	166	574		364
0.95	*	*	*	*	5	6	7	8	10	12	14	18	22	29	41	63	117	364	

* Sample size less than 5

Table 6h: Sample Size for Two-Sample Test of Proportions
(Level of significance: **10%**; Power: **80%**; Alternative hypothesis: **1-sided**)

P_1

P_2	0.05	0.10	0.15	0.20	0.25	0.30	0.35	0.40	0.45	0.50	0.55	0.60	0.65	0.70	0.75	0.80	0.85	0.90	0.95
0.10	250		394	115	57	36	25	18	14	11	9	8	7	6	5	*	*	*	*
0.15	81	394		521	144	70	42	28	21	16	12	10	8	7	6	5	*	*	*
0.20	43	115	521		629	169	80	47	31	22	17	13	10	8	7	6	5	*	*
0.25	28	57	144	629		719	189	88	51	33	24	18	14	11	9	7	6	5	*
0.30	20	36	70	169	719		791	205	94	54	35	24	18	14	11	8	7	6	5
0.35	16	25	42	80	189	791		845	216	98	55	36	25	18	14	10	8	7	5
0.40	12	18	28	47	88	205	845		882	223	100	56	36	24	18	13	10	8	6
0.45	10	14	21	31	51	94	216	882		900	225	100	55	35	24	17	12	9	7
0.50	8	11	16	22	33	54	98	223	900		900	223	98	54	33	22	16	11	8
0.55	7	9	12	17	24	35	55	100	225	900		882	216	94	51	31	21	14	10
0.60	6	8	10	13	18	24	36	56	100	223	882		845	205	88	47	28	18	12
0.65	5	7	8	10	14	18	25	36	55	98	216	845		791	189	80	42	25	16
0.70	5	6	7	8	11	14	18	24	35	54	94	205	791		719	169	70	36	20
0.75	*	5	6	7	9	11	14	18	24	33	51	88	189	719		629	144	57	28
0.80	*	*	5	6	7	8	10	13	17	22	31	47	80	169	629		521	115	43
0.85	*	*	*	5	6	7	8	10	12	16	21	28	42	70	144	521		394	81
0.90	*	*	*	*	5	6	7	8	9	11	14	18	25	36	57	115	394		250
0.95	*	*	*	*	*	5	5	6	7	8	10	12	16	20	28	43	81	250	

* Sample size less than 5

Table 6i: Sample Size for Two-Sample Test of Proportions
(Level of significance: **10%**; Power: **50%**; Alternative hypothesis: **1-sided**)

P₂	\(P_1\)																		
	0.05	0.10	0.15	0.20	0.25	0.30	0.35	0.40	0.45	0.50	0.55	0.60	0.65	0.70	0.75	0.80	0.85	0.90	0.95
0.10	92	144	144	42	22	14	10	7	6	5	*	*	*	*	*	*	*	*	*
0.15	30	144	190	190	53	26	16	11	8	6	5	*	*	*	*	*	*	*	*
0.20	16	42	190	230	230	62	30	18	12	9	7	5	*	*	*	*	*	*	*
0.25	11	22	53	230	263	263	70	33	19	13	9	7	5	*	*	*	*	*	*
0.30	8	14	26	62	263	289	289	75	35	20	13	9	7	6	*	*	*	*	*
0.35	6	10	16	30	70	289	309	309	79	37	21	14	10	7	5	*	*	*	*
0.40	5	7	11	18	33	75	309	322	322	82	37	21	14	9	7	5	*	*	*
0.45	*	6	8	12	19	35	79	322	328	328	83	37	21	13	9	7	5	*	*
0.50	*	5	6	9	13	20	37	82	328	328	328	82	37	20	13	9	6	5	*
0.55	*	*	5	7	9	13	21	37	83	328	328	322	79	35	19	12	8	6	*
0.60	*	*	*	5	7	9	14	21	37	82	322	322	309	75	33	18	11	7	5
0.65	*	*	*	*	5	7	10	14	21	37	79	309	309	289	70	30	16	10	6
0.70	*	*	*	*	*	6	7	9	13	20	35	75	289	289	263	62	26	14	8
0.75	*	*	*	*	*	*	5	7	9	13	19	33	70	263	263	230	53	22	11
0.80	*	*	*	*	*	*	*	5	7	9	12	18	30	62	230	230	190	42	16
0.85	*	*	*	*	*	*	*	*	5	6	8	11	16	26	53	190	190	144	30
0.90	*	*	*	*	*	*	*	*	*	5	6	7	10	14	22	42	144	144	92
0.95	*	*	*	*	*	*	*	*	*	*	*	5	6	8	11	16	30	92	92

* Sample size less than 5

Table 7a: Sample Size for Two-Sample Test of Proportions
(Level of significance: **1%**; Power: **90%**; Alternative hypothesis: **2-sided**)

The *smallest* of P_1, $(1-P_1)$, P_2 and $(1-P_2)$

$\lvert P_2 - P_1 \rvert$	0.05	0.10	0.15	0.20	0.25	0.30	0.35	0.40	0.45	0.50
0.01	15470	27973	38987	48513	56550	63099	68160	71732	73816	74411
0.02	4195	7284	10000	12344	14317	15917	17145	18000	18484	18596
0.03	2008	3364	4555	5580	6440	7135	7664	8028	8226	8260
0.04	1209	1963	2623	3191	3665	4047	4335	4530	4633	4642
0.05	824	1300	1717	2074	2372	2610	2789	2908	2967	2967
0.10	266	378	474	556	623	675	712	735	742	735
0.15	143	189	229	262	288	308	321	328	328	321
0.20	93	117	138	154	167	177	182	184	182	177
0.25	67	81	93	102	110	114	117	117	114	110
0.30	51	60	67	73	77	80	81	80	77	73
0.35	40	46	51	55	57	59	59	57	55	51
0.40	33	37	40	43	44	44	44	43	40	37
0.45	27	30	32	34	35	35	34	32	30	27
0.50	23	25	26	27	28	27	26	25	23	20

Table 7b: Sample Size for Two-Sample Test of Proportions
(Level of significance: **1%**;   Power: **80%**;   Alternative hypothesis: **2-sided**)

The *smallest* of P_1, $(1-P_1)$, P_2 and $(1-P_2)$

$|P_2-P_1|$	0.05	0.10	0.15	0.20	0.25	0.30	0.35	0.40	0.45	0.50
0.01	12143	21957	30602	38079	44388	49528	53500	56304	57940	58407
0.02	3294	5718	7850	9690	11238	12494	13458	14129	14509	14597
0.03	1577	2641	3576	4381	5056	5601	6016	6302	6458	6484
0.04	950	1541	2060	2505	2877	3177	3403	3556	3637	3644
0.05	647	1021	1348	1629	1862	2049	2190	2283	2330	2330
0.10	209	297	373	437	490	531	560	577	583	577
0.15	113	149	180	206	227	242	253	258	258	253
0.20	74	93	109	122	132	139	144	145	144	139
0.25	53	64	74	81	87	90	92	92	90	87
0.30	41	48	54	58	61	63	64	63	61	58
0.35	32	37	41	44	46	47	47	46	44	41
0.40	26	30	32	34	35	36	35	34	32	30
0.45	22	24	26	27	28	28	27	26	24	22
0.50	19	20	21	22	22	22	21	20	19	16

Table 7c: Sample Size for Two-Sample Test of Proportions
(Level of significance: **1%**; Power: **50%**; Alternative hypothesis: **2-sided**)

The *smallest* of P_1, $(1-P_1)$, P_2 and $(1-P_2)$

$|P_2-P_1|$	0.05	0.10	0.15	0.20	0.25	0.30	0.35	0.40	0.45	0.50
0.01	6898	12472	17383	21630	25213	28133	30389	31982	32911	33176
0.02	1872	3249	4460	5505	6384	7097	7645	8026	8242	8292
0.03	897	1501	2032	2489	2873	3182	3418	3581	3669	3684
0.04	540	876	1171	1424	1635	1805	1934	2021	2067	2071
0.05	369	581	767	926	1059	1165	1245	1298	1324	1324
0.10	120	170	213	249	279	302	319	329	332	329
0.15	65	86	103	118	130	139	145	148	148	145
0.20	43	54	63	70	76	80	83	83	83	80
0.25	31	38	43	47	50	52	53	53	52	50
0.30	24	28	31	34	36	37	37	37	36	34
0.35	19	22	24	26	27	28	28	27	26	24
0.40	16	18	19	20	21	21	21	20	19	18
0.45	14	15	16	17	17	17	17	16	15	14
0.50	12	13	13	14	14	14	13	13	12	10

Table 7d: Sample Size for Two-Sample Test of Proportions
(Level of significance: **5%**; Power: **90%**; Alternative hypothesis: **2-sided**)

The *smallest* of P_1, $(1-P_1)$, P_2 and $(1-P_2)$

$|P_2-P_1|$	0.05	0.10	0.15	0.20	0.25	0.30	0.35	0.40	0.45	0.50
0.01	10924	19753	27531	34258	39933	44558	48132	50654	52126	52546
0.02	2962	5143	7062	8717	10110	11239	12107	12711	13053	13131
0.03	1418	2376	3216	3940	4548	5038	5412	5669	5809	5832
0.04	854	1386	1852	2253	2588	2857	3061	3199	3271	3278
0.05	582	918	1212	1465	1675	1843	1969	2053	2095	2095
0.10	188	266	335	393	440	477	503	519	524	519
0.15	101	133	161	185	203	217	227	231	231	227
0.20	65	82	97	109	118	125	128	130	128	125
0.25	47	57	65	72	77	81	82	82	81	77
0.30	36	42	47	52	54	56	57	56	54	52
0.35	28	33	36	39	40	41	41	40	39	36
0.40	23	26	28	30	31	31	31	30	28	26
0.45	19	21	23	24	24	24	24	23	21	19
0.50	16	17	19	19	19	19	19	17	16	14

Table 7e: Sample Size for Two-Sample Test of Proportions
(Level of significance: **5%**; Power: **80%**; Alternative hypothesis: **2-sided**)

The *smallest* of P_1, $(1-P_1)$, P_2 and $(1-P_2)$

$|P_2-P_1|$	0.05	0.10	0.15	0.20	0.25	0.30	0.35	0.40	0.45	0.50
0.01	8161	14756	20566	25590	29830	33284	35954	37838	38937	39251
0.02	2213	3842	5275	6512	7552	8396	9044	9495	9751	9809
0.03	1060	1775	2403	2944	3398	3764	4043	4235	4340	4357
0.04	638	1036	1384	1683	1934	2135	2287	2390	2444	2449
0.05	435	686	906	1095	1252	1377	1471	1534	1566	1566
0.10	141	200	251	294	329	357	376	388	392	388
0.15	76	100	121	138	152	163	170	173	173	170
0.20	49	62	73	82	89	94	96	97	96	94
0.25	36	43	49	54	58	61	62	62	61	58
0.30	27	32	36	39	41	42	43	42	41	39
0.35	22	25	27	29	31	31	31	31	29	27
0.40	18	20	22	23	24	24	24	23	22	20
0.45	15	16	17	18	19	19	18	17	16	15
0.50	12	14	14	15	15	15	14	14	12	11

Table 7f: Sample Size for Two-Sample Test of Proportions
(Level of significance: **5%**; Power: **50%**; Alternative hypothesis: **2-sided**)

The *smallest* of P_1, $(1-P_1)$, P_2 and $(1-P_2)$

$|P_2-P_1|$	0.05	0.10	0.15	0.20	0.25	0.30	0.35	0.40	0.45	0.50
0.01	3994	7221	10064	12522	14597	16287	17593	18515	19053	19207
0.02	1084	1881	2582	3187	3696	4109	4426	4647	4772	4801
0.03	519	869	1177	1441	1663	1843	1979	2073	2124	2133
0.04	313	508	678	825	947	1045	1120	1170	1197	1199
0.05	214	337	444	536	613	675	721	752	767	767
0.10	70	98	123	145	162	175	185	191	193	191
0.15	38	50	60	69	75	81	84	86	86	84
0.20	25	31	37	41	44	47	48	49	48	47
0.25	18	22	25	27	29	31	31	31	31	29
0.30	14	17	18	20	21	22	22	22	21	20
0.35	11	13	14	15	16	16	16	16	15	14
0.40	10	11	11	12	12	13	12	12	11	11
0.45	8	9	9	10	10	10	10	9	9	8
0.50	7	7	8	8	8	8	8	7	7	6

Table 7g: Sample Size for Two-Sample Test of Proportions
(Level of significance: **10%**; Power: **90%**; Alternative hypothesis: **2-sided**)

The *smallest* of P_1, $(1-P_1)$, P_2 and $(1-P_2)$

$|P_2-P_1|$	0.05	0.10	0.15	0.20	0.25	0.30	0.35	0.40	0.45	0.50
0.01	8904	16101	22441	27924	32550	36320	39233	41289	42488	42831
0.02	2415	4192	5756	7105	8240	9161	9868	10361	10639	10704
0.03	1156	1936	2622	3212	3707	4107	4411	4621	4735	4754
0.04	696	1130	1510	1836	2109	2329	2495	2607	2666	2672
0.05	474	748	988	1194	1365	1502	1605	1674	1708	1708
0.10	153	217	273	320	358	388	410	423	427	423
0.15	82	109	131	150	166	177	185	189	189	185
0.20	53	67	79	89	96	101	105	106	105	101
0.25	38	46	53	59	63	66	67	67	66	63
0.30	29	34	39	42	44	46	46	46	44	42
0.35	23	26	29	31	33	33	33	33	31	29
0.40	19	21	23	24	25	25	25	24	23	21
0.45	15	17	18	19	20	20	19	18	17	15
0.50	13	14	15	16	16	16	15	14	13	11

Table 7h: Sample Size for Two-Sample Test of Proportions
(Level of significance: **10%**; Power: **80%**; Alternative hypothesis: **2-sided**)

The *smallest* of P_1, $(1-P_1)$, P_2 and $(1-P_2)$

$|P_2-P_1|$	0.05	0.10	0.15	0.20	0.25	0.30	0.35	0.40	0.45	0.50
0.01	6429	11624	16202	20160	23500	26221	28324	29809	30675	30922
0.02	1744	3027	4156	5130	5950	6614	7125	7480	7681	7728
0.03	835	1398	1893	2319	2677	2965	3185	3336	3419	3433
0.04	503	816	1090	1326	1523	1682	1802	1883	1925	1929
0.05	343	541	714	862	986	1085	1159	1209	1233	1233
0.10	111	157	197	231	259	281	296	306	309	306
0.15	60	79	95	109	120	128	134	137	137	134
0.20	39	49	57	64	70	74	76	77	76	74
0.25	28	34	39	43	46	48	49	49	48	46
0.30	21	25	28	31	32	33	34	33	32	31
0.35	17	20	22	23	24	25	25	24	23	22
0.40	14	16	17	18	19	19	19	18	17	16
0.45	12	13	14	14	15	15	14	14	13	12
0.50	10	11	11	12	12	12	11	11	10	9

Table 7i: Sample Size for Two-Sample Test of Proportions
(Level of significance: **10%**; Power: **50%**; Alternative hypothesis: **2-sided**)

The *smallest* of P_1, $(1-P_1)$, P_2 and $(1-P_2)$

$|P_2-P_1|$	0.05	0.10	0.15	0.20	0.25	0.30	0.35	0.40	0.45	0.50
0.01	2813	5086	7089	8821	10282	11473	12393	13042	13421	13529
0.02	764	1325	1819	2245	2604	2895	3118	3273	3361	3382
0.03	366	613	829	1015	1172	1298	1394	1460	1496	1502
0.04	221	358	478	581	667	737	789	824	843	845
0.05	151	237	313	378	432	475	508	530	540	540
0.10	49	70	87	102	114	124	130	134	136	134
0.15	27	35	42	48	53	57	59	60	60	59
0.20	18	22	26	29	31	33	34	34	34	33
0.25	13	16	18	19	21	22	22	22	22	21
0.30	10	12	13	14	15	15	16	15	15	14
0.35	8	9	10	11	11	12	12	11	11	10
0.40	7	8	8	9	9	9	9	9	8	8
0.45	6	6	7	7	7	7	7	7	6	6
0.50	5	5	6	6	6	6	6	5	5	5

Table 8a: Sample Size for Two-Sample Test of Small Proportions
(Level of significance: **1%**; Power: **90%**; Alternative hypothesis: **1-sided**)

P_1

P_2	0.0001	0.0002	0.0003	0.0004	0.0005	0.0010	0.0025	0.0050	0.0075	0.0100	0.0200	0.0300	0.0400
0.0001		379307	121433	65073	42589	13915	4064	1763	1106	801	374	242	178
0.0002	379307		644148	189625	96331	21289	5056	2030	1236	880	399	254	186
0.0003	121433	644148		906247	256118	31800	6087	2278	1352	948	419	265	192
0.0004	65073	189625	906247		1167438	48149	7223	2525	1463	1013	438	274	198
0.0005	42589	96331	256118	1167438		75817	8508	2778	1572	1075	456	283	203
0.0010	13915	21289	31800	48149	75817		19240	4248	2145	1386	535	321	226
0.0025	4064	5056	6087	7223	8508	19240		15119	4835	2588	771	423	284
0.0050	1763	2030	2278	2525	2778	4248	15119		25612	7531	1287	610	382
0.0075	1106	1236	1352	1463	1572	2145	4835	25612		35946	2137	853	495
0.0100	801	880	948	1013	1075	1386	2588	7531	35946		3738	1191	636
0.0200	374	399	419	438	456	535	771	1287	2137	3738		6283	1841
0.0300	242	254	265	274	283	321	423	610	853	1191	6283		8749
0.0400	178	186	192	198	203	226	284	382	495	636	1841	8749	
0.0500	140	146	150	154	158	173	211	272	338	414	931	2461	11155

Table 8b: Sample Size for Two-Sample Test of Small Proportions

(Level of significance: **1%**; Power: **80%**; Alternative hypothesis: **1-sided**)

P_2	\multicolumn{13}{c}{P_1}
	0.0001	0.0002	0.0003	0.0004	0.0005	0.0010	0.0025	0.0050	0.0075	0.0100	0.0200	0.0300	0.0400
0.0001		292434	93621	50169	32835	10728	3133	1359	853	617	288	186	137
0.0002	292434		496619	146195	74268	16413	3898	1565	953	678	307	196	143
0.0003	93621	496619		698689	197459	24517	4693	1757	1042	731	323	204	148
0.0004	50169	146195	698689		900059	37122	5568	1947	1128	781	338	211	153
0.0005	32835	74268	197459	900059		58452	6560	2142	1212	829	351	218	157
0.0010	10728	16413	24517	37122	58452		14834	3275	1654	1068	413	247	174
0.0025	3133	3898	4693	5568	6560	14834		11656	3728	1996	594	326	219
0.0050	1359	1565	1757	1947	2142	3275	11656		19746	5806	992	470	294
0.0075	853	953	1042	1128	1212	1654	3728	19746		27714	1648	657	382
0.0100	617	678	731	781	829	1068	1996	5806	27714		2882	918	490
0.0200	288	307	323	338	351	413	594	992	1648	2882		4844	1419
0.0300	186	196	204	211	218	247	326	470	657	918	4844		6745
0.0400	137	143	148	153	157	174	219	294	382	490	1419	6745	
0.0500	108	112	116	119	122	133	163	210	260	319	718	1897	8600

Table 8c: Sample Size for Two-Sample Test of Small Proportions
(Level of significance: **1%**; Power: **50%**; Alternative hypothesis: **1-sided**)

P_1

P_2	0.0001	0.0002	0.0003	0.0004	0.0005	0.0010	0.0025	0.0050	0.0075	0.0100	0.0200	0.0300	0.0400
0.0001		157644	50469	27045	17700	5783	1689	733	460	333	155	100	74
0.0002	157644		267715	78810	40036	8848	2101	844	514	366	166	106	77
0.0003	50469	267715		376646	106445	13216	2530	947	562	394	174	110	80
0.0004	27045	78810	376646		485199	20011	3002	1050	608	421	182	114	82
0.0005	17700	40036	106445	485199		31510	3536	1154	653	447	189	118	84
0.0010	5783	8848	13216	20011	31510		7996	1766	892	576	222	133	94
0.0025	1689	2101	2530	3002	3536	7996		6283	2009	1076	320	176	118
0.0050	733	844	947	1050	1154	1766	6283		10645	3130	535	253	159
0.0075	460	514	562	608	653	892	2009	10645		14940	888	354	206
0.0100	333	366	394	421	447	576	1076	3130	14940		1553	495	264
0.0200	155	166	174	182	189	222	320	535	888	1553		2611	765
0.0300	100	106	110	114	118	133	176	253	354	495	2611		3636
0.0400	74	77	80	82	84	94	118	159	206	264	765	3636	
0.0500	58	61	62	64	66	72	88	113	140	172	387	1023	4636

Table 8d: Sample Size for Two-Sample Test of Small Proportions
(Level of significance: **5%**;   Power: **90%**;   Alternative hypothesis: **1-sided**)

P_1

P_2	0.0001	0.0002	0.0003	0.0004	0.0005	0.0010	0.0025	0.0050	0.0075	0.0100	0.0200	0.0300	0.0400
0.0001		249634	79919	42827	28029	9158	2675	1160	728	527	246	159	117
0.0002	249634		423934	124798	63398	14011	3328	1336	813	579	262	167	122
0.0003	79919	423934		596429	168559	20928	4006	1500	890	624	276	174	126
0.0004	42827	124798	596429		768327	31688	4753	1662	963	667	288	180	130
0.0005	28029	63398	168559	768327		49897	5600	1828	1035	708	300	186	134
0.0010	9158	14011	20928	31688	49897		12662	2796	1412	912	352	211	149
0.0025	2675	3328	4006	4753	5600	12662		9950	3182	1703	507	278	187
0.0050	1160	1336	1500	1662	1828	2796	9950		16856	4957	847	401	251
0.0075	728	813	890	963	1035	1412	3182	16856		23657	1407	561	326
0.0100	527	579	624	667	708	912	1703	4957	23657		2460	784	418
0.0200	246	262	276	288	300	352	507	847	1407	2460		4135	1212
0.0300	159	167	174	180	186	211	278	401	561	784	4135		5758
0.0400	117	122	126	130	134	149	187	251	326	418	1212	5758	
0.0500	92	96	99	101	104	114	139	179	222	273	613	1619	7341

Table 8e: Sample Size for Two-Sample Test of Small Proportions
(Level of significance: **5%**; Power: **80%**; Alternative hypothesis: **1-sided**)

P_1

P_2	0.0001	0.0002	0.0003	0.0004	0.0005	0.0010	0.0025	0.0050	0.0075	0.0100	0.0200	0.0300	0.0400
0.0001		180223	57697	30919	20236	6611	1931	837	526	380	178	115	84
0.0002	180223		306058	90098	45770	10115	2402	964	587	418	189	121	88
0.0003	57697	306058		430591	121691	15109	2892	1083	642	451	199	126	91
0.0004	30919	90098	430591		554693	22877	3432	1200	695	481	208	130	94
0.0005	20236	45770	121691	554693		36023	4043	1320	747	511	216	134	97
0.0010	6611	10115	15109	22877	36023		9142	2019	1019	658	254	152	107
0.0025	1931	2402	2892	3432	4043	9142		7183	2297	1230	366	201	135
0.0050	837	964	1083	1200	1320	2019	7183		12169	3578	611	290	181
0.0075	526	587	642	695	747	1019	2297	12169		17079	1015	405	235
0.0100	380	418	451	481	511	658	1230	3578	17079		1776	566	302
0.0200	178	189	199	208	216	254	366	611	1015	1776		2985	875
0.0300	115	121	126	130	134	152	201	290	405	566	2985		4157
0.0400	84	88	91	94	97	107	135	181	235	302	875	4157	
0.0500	67	69	71	73	75	82	100	129	161	197	442	1169	5300

Table 8f: Sample Size for Two-Sample Test of Small Proportions
(Level of significance: **5%**; Power: **50%**; Alternative hypothesis: **1-sided**)

P_1

P_2	0.0001	0.0002	0.0003	0.0004	0.0005	0.0010	0.0025	0.0050	0.0075	0.0100	0.0200	0.0300	0.0400
0.0001		78848	25243	13527	8853	2893	845	366	230	166	78	50	37
0.0002	78848		133901	39418	20025	4425	1051	422	257	183	83	53	39
0.0003	25243	133901		188385	53240	6610	1265	474	281	197	87	55	40
0.0004	13527	39418	188385		242679	10009	1501	525	304	211	91	57	41
0.0005	8853	20025	53240	242679		15760	1769	577	327	224	95	59	42
0.0010	2893	4425	6610	10009	15760		4000	883	446	288	111	67	47
0.0025	845	1051	1265	1501	1769	4000		3143	1005	538	160	88	59
0.0050	366	422	474	525	577	883	3143		5324	1566	267	127	79
0.0075	230	257	281	304	327	446	1005	5324		7472	444	177	103
0.0100	166	183	197	211	224	288	538	1566	7472		777	248	132
0.0200	78	83	87	91	95	111	160	267	444	777		1306	383
0.0300	50	53	55	57	59	67	88	127	177	248	1306		1819
0.0400	37	39	40	41	42	47	59	79	103	132	383	1819	
0.0500	29	30	31	32	33	36	44	57	70	86	194	512	2319

Table 8g: Sample Size for Two-Sample Test of Small Proportions
(Level of significance: **10%**; Power: **90%**; Alternative hypothesis: **1-sided**)

P_1

P_2	0.0001	0.0002	0.0003	0.0004	0.0005	0.0010	0.0025	0.0050	0.0075	0.0100	0.0200	0.0300	0.0400
0.0001		191555	61325	32863	21508	7027	2052	890	559	404	189	122	90
0.0002	191555		325303	95763	48648	10751	2554	1025	624	444	201	128	94
0.0003	61325	325303		457667	129343	16059	3074	1151	683	479	212	134	97
0.0004	32863	95763	457667		589572	24316	3648	1275	739	511	221	138	100
0.0005	21508	48648	129343	589572		38288	4297	1403	794	543	230	143	103
0.0010	7027	10751	16059	24316	38288		9717	2145	1083	700	270	162	114
0.0025	2052	2554	3074	3648	4297	9717		7635	2442	1307	389	214	144
0.0050	890	1025	1151	1275	1403	2145	7635		12935	3803	650	308	193
0.0075	559	624	683	739	794	1083	2442	12935		18153	1079	431	250
0.0100	404	444	479	511	543	700	1307	3803	18153		1888	602	321
0.0200	189	201	212	221	230	270	389	650	1079	1888		3173	930
0.0300	122	128	134	138	143	162	214	308	431	602	3173		4419
0.0400	90	94	97	100	103	114	144	193	250	321	930	4419	
0.0500	71	74	76	78	80	87	107	137	171	209	470	1243	5633

Table 8h: Sample Size for Two-Sample Test of Small Proportions
(Level of significance: **10%**; Power: **80%**; Alternative hypothesis: **1-sided**)

P_1

P_2	0.0001	0.0002	0.0003	0.0004	0.0005	0.0010	0.0025	0.0050	0.0075	0.0100	0.0200	0.0300	0.0400
0.0001		131452	42084	22552	14760	4822	1408	611	383	277	130	84	62
0.0002	131452		223235	65716	33384	7378	1752	703	428	305	138	88	64
0.0003	42084	223235		314067	88760	11021	2110	790	468	329	145	92	67
0.0004	22552	65716	314067		404585	16686	2503	875	507	351	152	95	69
0.0005	14760	33384	88760	404585		26275	2949	963	545	373	158	98	70
0.0010	4822	7378	11021	16686	26275		6668	1472	743	480	186	111	78
0.0025	1408	1752	2110	2503	2949	6668		5239	1676	897	267	147	98
0.0050	611	703	790	875	963	1472	5239		8876	2610	446	211	132
0.0075	383	428	468	507	545	743	1676	8876		12457	741	295	172
0.0100	277	305	329	351	373	480	897	2610	12457		1295	413	220
0.0200	130	138	145	152	158	186	267	446	741	1295		2177	638
0.0300	84	88	92	95	98	111	147	211	295	413	2177		3032
0.0400	62	64	67	69	70	78	98	132	172	220	638	3032	
0.0500	49	50	52	53	55	60	73	94	117	144	323	853	3866

Table 8i: Sample Size for Two-Sample Test of Small Proportions
(Level of significance: **10%**; Power: **50%**; Alternative hypothesis: **1-sided**)

P_1

P_2	0.0001	0.0002	0.0003	0.0004	0.0005	0.0010	0.0025	0.0050	0.0075	0.0100	0.0200	0.0300	0.0400
0.0001		47889	15331	8216	5377	1757	513	223	140	101	47	31	22
0.0002	47889		81326	23941	12162	2688	638	256	156	111	50	32	23
0.0003	15331	81326		114417	32336	4015	769	288	171	120	53	33	24
0.0004	8216	23941	114417		147393	6079	912	319	185	128	55	35	25
0.0005	5377	12162	32336	147393		9572	1074	351	198	136	58	36	26
0.0010	1757	2688	4015	6079	9572		2429	536	271	175	68	40	29
0.0025	513	638	769	912	1074	2429		1909	610	327	97	53	36
0.0050	223	256	288	319	351	536	1909		3234	951	162	77	48
0.0075	140	156	171	185	198	271	610	3234		4538	270	108	63
0.0100	101	111	120	128	136	175	327	951	4538		472	150	80
0.0200	47	50	53	55	58	68	97	162	270	472		793	232
0.0300	31	32	33	35	36	40	53	77	108	150	793		1105
0.0400	22	23	24	25	26	29	36	48	63	80	232	1105	
0.0500	18	18	19	19	20	22	27	34	43	52	118	311	1408

Table 9a: Sample Size to Estimate the Odds Ratio to Within 10 % of True OR with **99%** Confidence

Odds Ratio (**OR**)

P*2	1.00	1.25	1.50	1.75	2.00	2.25	2.50	2.75	3.00	3.25	3.50	3.75	4.00	4.25	4.50	4.75	5.00
0.01	120763	108928	101039	95405	91179	87893	85264	83114	81322	79806	78507	77381	76396	75527	74755	74065	73443
0.02	60998	55143	51240	48454	46364	44740	43441	42379	41495	40747	40106	39551	39066	38638	38259	37919	37614
0.03	41085	37224	34651	32815	31439	30370	29515	28817	28236	27745	27325	26962	26644	26364	26116	25895	25696
0.04	31134	28271	26365	25005	23986	23195	22564	22048	21620	21258	20949	20682	20449	20245	20063	19902	19757
0.05	25170	22906	21400	20326	19522	18899	18402	17997	17661	17378	17136	16927	16746	16587	16446	16321	16210
0.10	13284	12225	11524	11028	10661	10378	10156	9977	9831	9709	9608	9522	9449	9386	9332	9286	9246
0.15	9377	8726	8301	8005	7789	7627	7503	7406	7330	7270	7221	7183	7153	7130	7112	7099	7089
0.20	7473	7032	6750	6560	6427	6331	6262	6213	6177	6154	6138	6130	6128	6130	6136	6145	6158
0.25	6377	6068	5879	5758	5679	5630	5600	5584	5580	5584	5594	5610	5630	5653	5679	5708	5739
0.30	5694	5479	5357	5288	5252	5239	5241	5254	5276	5304	5338	5375	5416	5460	5505	5553	5602
0.35	5256	5114	5047	5021	5022	5041	5072	5112	5159	5211	5267	5327	5389	5453	5519	5586	5655
0.40	4982	4902	4882	4897	4932	4982	5042	5109	5181	5258	5338	5420	5505	5591	5679	5768	5859
0.45	4831	4807	4832	4885	4955	5036	5126	5222	5322	5426	5532	5640	5750	5862	5975	6088	6203
0.50	4783	4813	4882	4975	5082	5198	5321	5448	5580	5714	5850	5988	6128	6268	6410	6552	6696
0.55	4831	4916	5033	5169	5317	5473	5633	5798	5966	6136	6308	6482	6656	6831	7008	7185	7362
0.60	4982	5126	5297	5484	5679	5881	6088	6297	6510	6724	6939	7156	7373	7591	7810	8030	8250
0.70	5694	5991	6306	6630	6960	7295	7632	7971	8312	8655	8998	9341	9686	10031	10376	10722	11068
0.80	7473	8041	8618	9202	9789	10378	10970	11562	12155	12749	13344	13939	14534	15129	15725	16321	16917
0.90	13284	14616	15952	17291	18631	19972	21314	22657	24000	25343	26687	28030	29374	30718	32063	33407	34751

Table 9b: Sample Size to Estimate the Odds Ratio to Within 20 % of True OR with **99%** Confidence

Odds Ratio (OR)

P^*_2	1.00	1.25	1.50	1.75	2.00	2.25	2.50	2.75	3.00	3.25	3.50	3.75	4.00	4.25	4.50	4.75	5.00
0.01	26923	24285	22526	21270	20328	19595	19009	18530	18130	17792	17503	17252	17032	16838	16666	16512	16374
0.02	13599	12294	11424	10803	10337	9975	9685	9448	9251	9084	8942	8818	8710	8614	8530	8454	8386
0.03	9160	8299	7725	7316	7009	6771	6581	6425	6295	6186	6092	6011	5940	5878	5823	5773	5729
0.04	6941	6303	5878	5575	5348	5172	5031	4916	4820	4740	4671	4611	4559	4514	4473	4437	4405
0.05	5612	5107	4771	4532	4353	4214	4103	4013	3938	3875	3821	3774	3734	3698	3667	3639	3614
0.10	2962	2726	2570	2459	2377	2314	2265	2225	2192	2165	2142	2123	2107	2093	2081	2071	2062
0.15	2091	1946	1851	1785	1737	1701	1673	1652	1635	1621	1610	1602	1595	1590	1586	1583	1581
0.20	1666	1568	1505	1463	1433	1412	1396	1385	1378	1372	1369	1367	1366	1367	1368	1370	1373
0.25	1422	1353	1311	1284	1267	1255	1249	1245	1244	1245	1247	1251	1255	1261	1267	1273	1280
0.30	1270	1222	1195	1179	1171	1168	1169	1172	1177	1183	1190	1199	1208	1218	1228	1238	1249
0.35	1172	1141	1125	1120	1120	1124	1131	1140	1151	1162	1175	1188	1202	1216	1231	1246	1261
0.40	1111	1093	1089	1092	1100	1111	1124	1139	1155	1173	1190	1209	1228	1247	1267	1286	1307
0.45	1077	1072	1078	1089	1105	1123	1143	1165	1187	1210	1234	1258	1282	1307	1332	1358	1383
0.50	1067	1073	1089	1109	1133	1159	1187	1215	1244	1274	1305	1335	1366	1398	1429	1461	1493
0.55	1077	1096	1123	1153	1186	1220	1256	1293	1330	1368	1407	1445	1484	1523	1563	1602	1642
0.60	1111	1143	1181	1223	1267	1312	1358	1404	1452	1499	1547	1596	1644	1693	1742	1791	1840
0.70	1270	1336	1406	1478	1552	1627	1702	1778	1854	1930	2006	2083	2160	2237	2314	2391	2468
0.80	1666	1793	1922	2052	2183	2314	2446	2578	2710	2843	2975	3108	3241	3373	3506	3639	3772
0.90	2962	3259	3557	3855	4154	4453	4752	5052	5351	5650	5950	6249	6549	6849	7148	7448	7748

Table 9c: Sample Size to Estimate the Odds Ratio to Within 25 % of True OR with 99% Confidence

Odds Ratio (OR)

P^*_2	1.00	1.25	1.50	1.75	2.00	2.25	2.50	2.75	3.00	3.25	3.50	3.75	4.00	4.25	4.50	4.75	5.00
0.01	16198	14611	13553	12797	12230	11790	11437	11149	10908	10705	10531	10380	10248	10131	10027	9935	9851
0.02	8182	7397	6873	6500	6219	6002	5827	5685	5566	5466	5380	5305	5240	5183	5132	5087	5046
0.03	5511	4993	4648	4402	4217	4074	3959	3866	3788	3722	3666	3617	3574	3537	3503	3474	3447
0.04	4177	3793	3537	3354	3218	3112	3027	2958	2900	2852	2810	2775	2743	2716	2692	2670	2650
0.05	3377	3073	2871	2727	2619	2535	2469	2414	2369	2331	2299	2271	2247	2225	2206	2190	2175
0.10	1782	1640	1546	1480	1430	1393	1363	1339	1319	1303	1289	1278	1268	1259	1252	1246	1241
0.15	1258	1171	1114	1074	1045	1023	1007	994	984	976	969	964	960	957	954	953	951
0.20	1003	944	906	880	862	850	840	834	829	826	824	823	822	823	823	825	826
0.25	856	814	789	773	762	756	752	749	749	749	751	753	756	759	762	766	770
0.30	764	735	719	710	705	703	703	705	708	712	716	721	727	733	739	745	752
0.35	705	686	677	674	674	677	681	686	692	699	707	715	723	732	741	750	759
0.40	669	658	655	657	662	669	677	686	695	706	716	727	739	750	762	774	786
0.45	648	645	649	656	665	676	688	701	714	728	742	757	772	787	802	817	832
0.50	642	646	655	668	682	698	714	731	749	767	785	804	822	841	860	879	899
0.55	648	660	676	694	714	734	756	778	801	823	847	870	893	917	940	964	988
0.60	669	688	711	736	762	789	817	845	874	902	931	960	989	1019	1048	1077	1107
0.70	764	804	846	890	934	979	1024	1070	1115	1161	1207	1253	1300	1346	1392	1439	1485
0.80	1003	1079	1156	1235	1313	1393	1472	1551	1631	1710	1790	1870	1950	2030	2110	2190	2270
0.90	1782	1961	2140	2320	2499	2679	2859	3039	3220	3400	3580	3760	3940	4121	4301	4481	4662

Table 9d: Sample Size to Estimate the Odds Ratio to Within 50 % of True OR with **99%** Confidence

Odds Ratio (OR)

P^*_2	1.00	1.25	1.50	1.75	2.00	2.25	2.50	2.75	3.00	3.25	3.50	3.75	4.00	4.25	4.50	4.75	5.00
0.01	2791	2517	2335	2205	2107	2031	1971	1921	1879	1844	1814	1788	1766	1746	1728	1712	1697
0.02	1410	1275	1184	1120	1072	1034	1004	980	959	942	927	914	903	893	884	877	870
0.03	950	861	801	759	727	702	682	666	653	642	632	623	616	610	604	599	594
0.04	720	654	610	578	555	536	522	510	500	492	485	478	473	468	464	460	457
0.05	582	530	495	470	452	437	426	416	409	402	396	392	387	384	380	378	375
0.10	307	283	267	255	247	240	235	231	228	225	222	220	219	217	216	215	214
0.15	217	202	192	185	180	177	174	172	170	168	167	166	166	165	165	165	164
0.20	173	163	156	152	149	147	145	144	143	143	142	142	142	142	142	142	143
0.25	148	141	136	134	132	131	130	130	129	129	130	130	131	131	132	132	133
0.30	132	127	124	123	122	122	122	122	122	123	124	125	126	127	128	129	130
0.35	122	119	117	117	117	117	118	119	120	121	122	124	125	126	128	130	131
0.40	116	114	113	114	114	116	117	119	120	122	124	126	128	130	132	134	136
0.45	112	112	112	113	115	117	119	121	123	126	128	131	133	136	139	141	144
0.50	111	112	113	115	118	121	123	126	129	133	136	139	142	145	149	152	155
0.55	112	114	117	120	123	127	131	134	138	142	146	150	154	158	162	166	171
0.60	116	119	123	127	132	136	141	146	151	156	161	166	171	176	181	186	191
0.70	132	139	146	154	161	169	177	185	193	200	208	216	224	232	240	248	256
0.80	173	186	200	213	227	240	254	268	281	295	309	323	336	350	364	378	391
0.90	307	338	369	400	431	462	493	524	555	586	617	648	679	710	741	772	803

Table 9e: Sample Size to Estimate the Odds Ratio to Within
10 % of True OR with **95%** Confidence

Odds Ratio (**OR**)

P^*_2	1.00	1.25	1.50	1.75	2.00	2.25	2.50	2.75	3.00	3.25	3.50	3.75	4.00	4.25	4.50	4.75	5.00
0.01	69912	63061	58494	55232	52786	50883	49361	48116	47079	46202	45449	44798	44228	43725	43278	42878	42518
0.02	35313	31923	29664	28051	26842	25901	25149	24535	24023	23589	23219	22897	22616	22369	22149	21952	21776
0.03	23785	21550	20061	18998	18201	17582	17087	16683	16347	16063	15819	15609	15425	15263	15120	14991	14876
0.04	18025	16367	15263	14476	13886	13429	13063	12765	12516	12307	12128	11974	11839	11720	11615	11522	11438
0.05	14572	13261	12389	11767	11302	10941	10654	10419	10225	10061	9921	9800	9695	9603	9521	9449	9384
0.10	7691	7078	6672	6385	6172	6009	5880	5776	5691	5621	5562	5513	5470	5434	5403	5376	5353
0.15	5429	5052	4806	4634	4510	4416	4344	4288	4244	4209	4181	4159	4141	4128	4117	4110	4104
0.20	4326	4071	3908	3798	3721	3665	3626	3597	3576	3563	3554	3549	3548	3549	3552	3558	3565
0.25	3692	3513	3403	3333	3288	3259	3242	3233	3230	3233	3239	3248	3259	3273	3288	3305	3323
0.30	3296	3172	3101	3062	3041	3033	3034	3042	3055	3071	3090	3112	3136	3161	3187	3215	3244
0.35	3043	2961	2922	2907	2908	2919	2937	2960	2987	3017	3050	3084	3120	3157	3195	3234	3274
0.40	2884	2838	2827	2835	2856	2884	2919	2958	3000	3044	3090	3138	3187	3237	3288	3340	3392
0.45	2797	2783	2798	2828	2869	2916	2968	3023	3081	3141	3203	3265	3329	3394	3459	3525	3591
0.50	2769	2786	2827	2880	2942	3009	3080	3154	3230	3308	3387	3467	3548	3629	3711	3794	3876
0.55	2797	2846	2914	2993	3078	3168	3262	3357	3454	3553	3652	3752	3854	3955	4057	4160	4262
0.60	2884	2968	3067	3175	3288	3405	3525	3646	3769	3893	4017	4143	4269	4395	4522	4649	4776
0.70	3296	3469	3651	3838	4030	4223	4419	4615	4812	5011	5209	5408	5608	5807	6007	6207	6408
0.80	4326	4655	4990	5327	5667	6009	6351	6694	7037	7381	7725	8070	8414	8759	9104	9449	9794
0.90	7691	8462	9235	10010	10786	11563	12340	13117	13894	14672	15450	16228	17006	17784	18562	19340	20118

Table 9f: Sample Size to Estimate the Odds Ratio to Within 20 % of True OR with **95%** Confidence

Odds Ratio (OR)

P^*_2	1.00	1.25	1.50	1.75	2.00	2.25	2.50	2.75	3.00	3.25	3.50	3.75	4.00	4.25	4.50	4.75	5.00
0.01	15587	14059	13041	12314	11768	11344	11005	10727	10496	10301	10133	9988	9860	9748	9649	9560	9479
0.02	7873	7117	6614	6254	5984	5775	5607	5470	5356	5259	5177	5105	5042	4987	4938	4894	4855
0.03	5303	4805	4473	4236	4058	3920	3810	3720	3645	3581	3527	3480	3439	3403	3371	3343	3317
0.04	4019	3649	3403	3228	3096	2994	2913	2846	2791	2744	2704	2670	2640	2613	2590	2569	2550
0.05	3249	2957	2762	2624	2520	2440	2376	2323	2280	2243	2212	2185	2162	2141	2123	2107	2093
0.10	1715	1578	1488	1424	1376	1340	1311	1288	1269	1254	1240	1229	1220	1212	1205	1199	1194
0.15	1211	1127	1072	1034	1006	985	969	956	946	939	932	928	924	921	918	917	915
0.20	965	908	872	847	830	818	809	802	798	795	793	792	791	792	792	794	795
0.25	823	784	759	744	733	727	723	721	721	721	722	724	727	730	733	737	741
0.30	735	708	692	683	678	677	677	679	681	685	689	694	699	705	711	717	724
0.35	679	660	652	649	649	651	655	660	666	673	680	688	696	704	713	721	730
0.40	643	633	631	632	637	643	651	660	669	679	689	700	711	722	733	745	757
0.45	624	621	624	631	640	650	662	674	687	701	714	728	743	757	772	786	801
0.50	618	622	631	643	656	671	687	704	721	738	755	773	791	809	828	846	865
0.55	624	635	650	668	687	707	728	749	770	792	815	837	859	882	905	928	951
0.60	643	662	684	708	733	760	786	813	841	868	896	924	952	980	1008	1037	1065
0.70	735	774	814	856	899	942	985	1029	1073	1117	1162	1206	1251	1295	1340	1384	1429
0.80	965	1038	1113	1188	1264	1340	1416	1493	1569	1646	1723	1799	1876	1953	2030	2107	2184
0.90	1715	1887	2059	2232	2405	2578	2751	2925	3098	3271	3445	3618	3792	3965	4139	4312	4486

Table 9g: Sample Size to Estimate the Odds Ratio to Within 25 % of True OR with **95%** Confidence

Odds Ratio (**OR**)

P*$_2$	1.00	1.25	1.50	1.75	2.00	2.25	2.50	2.75	3.00	3.25	3.50	3.75	4.00	4.25	4.50	4.75	5.00
0.01	9378	8459	7846	7409	7081	6825	6621	6454	6315	6198	6097	6009	5933	5865	5805	5752	5703
0.02	4737	4282	3979	3763	3601	3475	3374	3291	3223	3165	3115	3072	3034	3001	2971	2945	2921
0.03	3191	2891	2691	2549	2442	2359	2292	2238	2193	2155	2122	2094	2069	2048	2028	2011	1996
0.04	2418	2196	2048	1942	1863	1802	1753	1713	1679	1651	1627	1606	1588	1572	1558	1546	1535
0.05	1955	1779	1662	1579	1516	1468	1429	1398	1372	1350	1331	1315	1301	1288	1278	1268	1259
0.10	1032	950	895	857	828	806	789	775	764	754	747	740	734	729	725	722	718
0.15	729	678	645	622	605	593	583	576	570	565	561	558	556	554	553	552	551
0.20	581	546	525	510	499	492	487	483	480	478	477	476	476	476	477	478	479
0.25	496	472	457	448	441	438	435	434	434	434	435	436	438	439	441	444	446
0.30	443	426	416	411	408	407	407	408	410	412	415	418	421	424	428	432	436
0.35	409	398	392	390	390	392	394	397	401	405	409	414	419	424	429	434	440
0.40	387	381	380	381	383	387	392	397	403	409	415	421	428	435	441	448	455
0.45	376	374	376	380	385	392	399	406	414	422	430	438	447	456	464	473	482
0.50	372	374	380	387	395	404	414	424	434	444	455	465	476	487	498	509	520
0.55	376	382	391	402	413	425	438	451	464	477	490	504	517	531	545	558	572
0.60	387	399	412	426	441	457	473	489	506	523	539	556	573	590	607	624	641
0.70	443	466	490	515	541	567	593	619	646	672	699	726	753	779	806	833	860
0.80	581	625	670	715	761	806	852	898	944	990	1037	1083	1129	1175	1222	1268	1314
0.90	1032	1135	1239	1343	1447	1551	1656	1760	1864	1968	2073	2177	2281	2386	2490	2595	2699

Table 9h: Sample Size to Estimate the Odds Ratio to Within
50 % of True OR with **95%** Confidence

Odds Ratio (OR)

P^*_2	1.00	1.25	1.50	1.75	2.00	2.25	2.50	2.75	3.00	3.25	3.50	3.75	4.00	4.25	4.50	4.75	5.00
0.01	1616	1458	1352	1277	1220	1176	1141	1112	1088	1068	1051	1036	1022	1011	1000	991	983
0.02	816	738	686	649	621	599	582	567	556	546	537	530	523	517	512	508	504
0.03	550	498	464	439	421	407	395	386	378	372	366	361	357	353	350	347	344
0.04	417	379	353	335	321	311	302	295	290	285	281	277	274	271	269	267	265
0.05	337	307	287	272	262	253	247	241	237	233	230	227	224	222	220	219	217
0.10	178	164	155	148	143	139	136	134	132	130	129	128	127	126	125	125	124
0.15	126	117	112	108	105	103	101	100	99	98	97	97	96	96	96	95	95
0.20	100	95	91	88	86	85	84	84	83	83	83	82	82	82	83	83	83
0.25	86	82	79	78	76	76	75	75	75	75	75	76	76	76	76	77	77
0.30	77	74	72	71	71	71	71	71	71	71	72	72	73	74	74	75	75
0.35	71	69	68	68	68	68	68	69	70	70	71	72	73	73	74	75	76
0.40	67	66	66	66	66	67	68	69	70	71	72	73	74	75	76	78	79
0.45	65	65	65	66	67	68	69	70	72	73	74	76	77	79	80	82	83
0.50	64	65	66	67	68	70	72	73	75	77	79	81	82	84	86	88	90
0.55	65	66	68	70	72	74	76	78	80	83	85	87	90	92	94	97	99
0.60	67	69	71	74	76	79	82	85	88	90	93	96	99	102	105	108	111
0.70	77	81	85	89	94	98	103	107	112	116	121	125	130	135	139	144	149
0.80	100	108	116	124	131	139	147	155	163	171	179	187	195	203	211	219	227
0.90	178	196	214	232	250	268	286	304	322	339	357	375	393	411	429	447	465

Table 9i: Sample Size to Estimate the Odds Ratio to Within 10 % of True OR with **90%** Confidence

Odds Ratio (OR)

P_2^*	1.00	1.25	1.50	1.75	2.00	2.25	2.50	2.75	3.00	3.25	3.50	3.75	4.00	4.25	4.50	4.75	5.00
0.01	49246	44421	41203	38906	37182	35842	34770	33893	33163	32545	32015	31556	31154	30800	30485	30203	29950
0.02	24875	22487	20896	19759	18907	18245	17715	17282	16922	16617	16355	16129	15931	15757	15602	15463	15339
0.03	16754	15180	14131	13382	12821	12385	12037	11752	11515	11315	11143	10995	10866	10752	10650	10560	10479
0.04	12697	11529	10752	10197	9782	9459	9202	8992	8817	8669	8543	8434	8339	8256	8182	8116	8057
0.05	10264	9341	8727	8289	7961	7707	7505	7339	7202	7087	6988	6903	6829	6764	6707	6656	6610
0.10	5418	4986	4700	4498	4348	4233	4142	4069	4009	3960	3918	3883	3853	3828	3806	3787	3771
0.15	3824	3559	3385	3265	3177	3111	3060	3021	2989	2965	2945	2930	2917	2908	2900	2895	2891
0.20	3048	2868	2753	2675	2621	2582	2554	2534	2519	2510	2503	2500	2499	2500	2503	2506	2511
0.25	2601	2475	2398	2348	2316	2296	2284	2278	2276	2277	2281	2288	2296	2306	2316	2328	2341
0.30	2322	2234	2185	2157	2142	2137	2138	2143	2152	2163	2177	2192	2209	2227	2245	2265	2285
0.35	2144	2086	2058	2048	2048	2056	2069	2085	2104	2125	2148	2172	2198	2224	2251	2278	2306
0.40	2032	1999	1991	1997	2012	2032	2056	2084	2113	2144	2177	2211	2245	2280	2316	2353	2389
0.45	1970	1961	1971	1992	2021	2054	2091	2130	2171	2213	2256	2300	2345	2391	2437	2483	2530
0.50	1951	1963	1991	2029	2073	2120	2170	2222	2276	2330	2386	2442	2499	2556	2614	2672	2731
0.55	1970	2005	2053	2108	2169	2232	2298	2365	2433	2503	2573	2643	2715	2786	2858	2930	3003
0.60	2032	2091	2161	2236	2316	2399	2483	2568	2655	2742	2830	2918	3007	3096	3185	3275	3364
0.70	2322	2443	2572	2704	2839	2975	3113	3251	3390	3530	3669	3810	3950	4091	4232	4373	4514
0.80	3048	3279	3515	3753	3992	4233	4474	4715	4957	5199	5442	5684	5927	6170	6413	6656	6899
0.90	5418	5961	6505	7051	7598	8145	8692	9240	9787	10335	10883	11431	11979	12527	13075	13623	14172

Table 9j: Sample Size to Estimate the Odds Ratio to Within 20 % of True OR with **90%** Confidence

Odds Ratio (OR)

P^*_2	1.00	1.25	1.50	1.75	2.00	2.25	2.50	2.75	3.00	3.25	3.50	3.75	4.00	4.25	4.50	4.75	5.00
0.01	10979	9903	9186	8674	8290	7991	7752	7557	7394	7256	7138	7035	6946	6867	6797	6734	6677
0.02	5546	5014	4659	4406	4216	4068	3950	3853	3773	3705	3647	3596	3552	3513	3479	3448	3420
0.03	3736	3385	3151	2984	2859	2761	2684	2620	2567	2523	2485	2452	2423	2397	2375	2355	2337
0.04	2831	2571	2397	2274	2181	2109	2052	2005	1966	1933	1905	1881	1860	1841	1824	1810	1797
0.05	2289	2083	1946	1848	1775	1719	1673	1637	1606	1580	1558	1539	1523	1508	1496	1484	1474
0.10	1208	1112	1048	1003	970	944	924	907	894	883	874	866	859	854	849	845	841
0.15	853	794	755	728	709	694	683	674	667	661	657	654	651	649	647	646	645
0.20	680	640	614	597	585	576	570	565	562	560	559	558	558	558	558	559	560
0.25	580	552	535	524	517	512	510	508	508	508	509	510	512	514	517	519	522
0.30	518	499	487	481	478	477	477	478	480	483	486	489	493	497	501	505	510
0.35	478	465	459	457	457	459	462	465	470	474	479	485	490	496	502	508	515
0.40	453	446	444	446	449	453	459	465	471	478	486	493	501	509	517	525	533
0.45	440	437	440	445	451	458	466	475	484	494	503	513	523	533	544	554	564
0.50	435	438	444	453	462	473	484	496	508	520	532	545	558	570	583	596	609
0.55	440	447	458	470	484	498	513	528	543	558	574	590	606	622	638	654	670
0.60	453	467	482	499	517	535	554	573	592	612	631	651	671	691	711	730	750
0.70	518	545	574	603	633	664	694	725	756	787	818	850	881	912	944	975	1007
0.80	680	731	784	837	890	944	998	1052	1106	1160	1214	1268	1322	1376	1430	1484	1538
0.90	1208	1329	1451	1572	1694	1816	1938	2060	2182	2304	2427	2549	2671	2793	2915	3038	3160

Table 9k: Sample Size to Estimate the Odds Ratio to Within 25 % of True OR with 90% Confidence

Odds Ratio (OR)

P^*_2	1.00	1.25	1.50	1.75	2.00	2.25	2.50	2.75	3.00	3.25	3.50	3.75	4.00	4.25	4.50	4.75	5.00
0.01	6606	5959	5527	5219	4988	4808	4664	4547	4449	4366	4295	4233	4179	4132	4089	4052	4018
0.02	3337	3017	2803	2651	2537	2448	2377	2319	2270	2229	2194	2164	2137	2114	2093	2075	2058
0.03	2248	2037	1896	1795	1720	1662	1615	1577	1545	1518	1495	1475	1458	1443	1429	1417	1406
0.04	1703	1547	1443	1368	1312	1269	1235	1206	1183	1163	1146	1132	1119	1108	1098	1089	1081
0.05	1377	1253	1171	1112	1068	1034	1007	985	966	951	938	926	916	908	900	893	887
0.10	727	669	631	604	584	568	556	546	538	532	526	521	517	514	511	508	506
0.15	513	478	455	438	427	418	411	406	401	398	395	393	392	390	389	389	388
0.20	409	385	370	359	352	347	343	340	338	337	336	336	336	336	336	337	337
0.25	349	332	322	315	311	308	307	306	306	306	306	307	308	310	311	313	314
0.30	312	300	293	290	288	287	287	288	289	291	292	294	297	299	302	304	307
0.35	288	280	277	275	275	276	278	280	283	286	289	292	295	299	302	306	310
0.40	273	269	268	268	270	273	276	280	284	288	292	297	302	306	311	316	321
0.45	265	263	265	268	271	276	281	286	292	297	303	309	315	321	327	333	340
0.50	262	264	268	273	278	285	292	298	306	313	320	328	336	343	351	359	367
0.55	265	269	276	283	291	300	309	318	327	336	346	355	365	374	384	393	403
0.60	273	281	290	300	311	322	333	345	357	368	380	392	404	416	428	440	452
0.70	312	328	345	363	381	399	418	436	455	474	493	511	530	549	568	587	606
0.80	409	440	472	504	536	568	600	633	665	698	730	763	795	828	861	893	926
0.90	727	800	873	946	1020	1093	1166	1240	1313	1387	1460	1534	1607	1681	1754	1828	1901

Table 9I: Sample Size to Estimate the Odds Ratio to Within
50 % of True OR with **90%** Confidence

Odds Ratio (**OR**)

P^*_2	1.00	1.25	1.50	1.75	2.00	2.25	2.50	2.75	3.00	3.25	3.50	3.75	4.00	4.25	4.50	4.75	5.00
0.01	1138	1027	952	899	860	829	804	784	767	752	740	730	720	712	705	698	692
0.02	575	520	483	457	437	422	410	400	391	384	378	373	369	365	361	358	355
0.03	388	351	327	310	297	287	279	272	267	262	258	255	252	249	247	244	243
0.04	294	267	249	236	226	219	213	208	204	201	198	195	193	191	190	188	187
0.05	238	216	202	192	184	179	174	170	167	164	162	160	158	157	155	154	153
0.10	126	116	109	104	101	98	96	94	93	92	91	90	90	89	88	88	88
0.15	89	83	79	76	74	72	71	70	70	69	69	68	68	68	68	67	67
0.20	71	67	64	62	61	60	59	59	59	58	58	58	58	58	58	58	59
0.25	61	58	56	55	54	54	53	53	53	53	53	53	54	54	54	54	55
0.30	54	52	51	50	50	50	50	50	50	50	51	51	52	52	52	53	53
0.35	50	49	48	48	48	48	48	49	49	50	50	51	51	52	52	53	54
0.40	47	47	46	47	47	47	48	49	49	50	51	52	52	53	54	55	56
0.45	46	46	46	47	47	48	49	49	51	52	53	54	55	56	57	58	59
0.50	46	46	46	47	48	49	51	52	53	54	56	57	58	60	61	62	64
0.55	46	47	48	49	51	52	54	55	57	58	60	62	63	65	67	68	70
0.60	47	49	50	52	54	56	58	60	62	64	66	68	70	72	74	76	78
0.70	54	57	60	63	66	69	72	76	79	82	85	89	92	95	98	102	105
0.80	71	76	82	87	93	98	104	109	115	121	126	132	137	143	149	154	160
0.90	126	138	151	163	176	189	201	214	227	239	252	265	277	290	303	315	328

Table 10a: Sample Size for a Hypothesis Test of the Odds Ratio
(Level of significance: **1%**; Power: **90%**; Alternative hypothesis: **2-sided**)

Odds Ratio (**OR**)

P*$_2$	1.25	1.50	1.75	2.00	2.25	2.50	2.75	3.00	3.25	3.50	3.75	4.00	4.25	4.50	4.75	5.00
0.01	50273	13092	6046	3525	2334	1674	1269	1000	813	677	574	495	432	381	340	305
0.02	25496	6665	3089	1808	1201	864	657	519	423	353	301	260	227	201	180	162
0.03	17242	4524	2104	1236	824	595	453	360	294	246	210	182	160	142	127	115
0.04	13119	3456	1613	950	635	460	352	280	229	193	165	143	126	112	101	91
0.05	10648	2815	1319	780	523	380	291	232	191	161	138	120	106	94	85	77
0.10	5733	1544	736	442	301	222	173	139	116	99	86	75	67	61	55	50
0.15	4128	1132	548	335	231	173	136	111	94	81	71	63	56	51	47	43
0.20	3355	936	461	285	200	151	120	99	84	73	65	58	53	48	45	41
0.25	2919	829	414	260	184	141	113	95	81	71	63	57	52	48	45	42
0.30	2657	767	389	247	177	137	111	94	81	72	64	58	54	50	46	44
0.35	2500	733	377	243	176	137	113	96	83	74	67	61	56	53	49	47
0.40	2415	720	375	244	179	141	117	100	87	78	71	65	61	57	53	51
0.45	2386	722	382	251	186	148	123	106	94	84	77	71	66	62	59	56
0.50	2407	740	396	263	197	158	132	115	102	92	84	78	73	69	65	62
0.55	2476	772	418	281	212	171	144	126	112	102	94	87	82	78	74	71
0.60	2601	823	451	306	233	189	161	141	126	115	106	99	94	89	85	81
0.70	3082	1003	562	389	300	247	212	188	170	156	145	136	129	123	118	114
0.80	4192	1401	801	564	441	367	319	284	259	240	224	212	202	193	186	179
0.90	7718	2646	1544	1102	873	735	643	578	530	493	464	440	421	404	390	378

Table 10b: Sample Size for a Hypothesis Test of the Odds Ratio
(Level of significance: **1%**;   Power: **80%**;   Alternative hypothesis: **2-sided**)

Odds Ratio (**OR**

P_2^*	1.25	1.50	1.75	2.00	2.25	2.50	2.75	3.00	3.25	3.50	3.75	4.00	4.25	4.50	4.75	5.00
0.01	39067	10082	4617	2672	1757	1252	943	739	598	495	418	358	312	274	243	218
0.02	19817	5135	2361	1372	905	647	489	385	312	259	220	189	165	145	129	116
0.03	13405	3488	1610	939	622	446	338	267	217	181	154	133	116	103	92	83
0.04	10202	2665	1235	723	481	346	263	209	170	142	121	105	92	82	73	66
0.05	8283	2173	1011	594	396	286	219	174	142	119	102	88	78	69	62	56
0.10	4465	1195	566	339	230	169	131	105	88	74	64	57	50	45	41	38
0.15	3218	878	424	257	177	132	104	85	71	61	54	48	43	39	36	33
0.20	2618	728	357	221	154	116	93	77	65	57	50	45	41	37	34	32
0.25	2281	646	322	202	143	109	88	73	63	55	49	44	41	37	35	33
0.30	2078	599	303	193	138	107	87	73	63	56	50	46	42	39	36	34
0.35	1957	574	295	190	138	108	88	75	65	58	53	48	45	42	39	37
0.40	1893	564	294	192	141	111	92	79	69	62	56	52	48	45	42	40
0.45	1872	567	300	198	147	117	97	84	74	67	61	56	53	50	47	45
0.50	1890	582	312	208	156	125	105	91	81	73	67	62	58	55	52	50
0.55	1947	608	330	223	168	136	115	100	90	82	75	70	66	62	59	57
0.60	2047	649	357	243	185	151	128	113	101	92	85	80	75	72	68	66
0.70	2429	794	446	309	239	198	170	151	137	126	117	110	105	100	96	92
0.80	3310	1112	638	450	353	295	256	229	209	194	182	172	164	157	151	146
0.90	6104	2105	1233	884	702	592	519	468	430	400	377	358	343	329	318	309

Table 10c: Sample Size for a Hypothesis Test of the Odds Ratio
(Level of significance: **1%**;   Power: **50%**;   Alternative hypothesis: **2-sided**)

Odds Ratio (OR)

P^*_2	1.25	1.50	1.75	2.00	2.25	2.50	2.75	3.00	3.25	3.50	3.75	4.00	4.25	4.50	4.75	5.00
0.01	21557	5416	2420	1368	880	614	454	349	277	226	188	159	136	118	103	91
0.02	10943	2763	1241	705	456	320	237	184	147	120	100	85	73	64	56	50
0.03	7407	1880	848	484	315	222	165	129	103	85	71	61	53	46	41	36
0.04	5641	1439	652	374	244	173	130	101	82	67	57	49	42	37	33	30
0.05	4583	1175	535	309	202	144	108	85	69	57	48	42	36	32	29	26
0.10	2479	651	303	179	120	87	67	54	44	37	32	28	25	22	20	19
0.15	1793	482	230	138	94	70	55	44	37	32	28	25	22	20	19	17
0.20	1464	402	196	120	83	63	50	41	35	30	27	24	22	20	19	17
0.25	1279	359	178	111	79	60	48	40	35	30	27	25	23	21	19	18
0.30	1169	335	169	107	77	60	48	41	36	31	28	26	24	22	21	20
0.35	1104	323	166	107	78	61	50	43	37	33	30	28	26	24	23	22
0.40	1071	319	167	109	80	63	53	45	40	36	33	30	28	27	25	24
0.45	1062	322	171	113	84	67	56	49	43	39	36	33	31	30	28	27
0.50	1075	332	179	120	90	73	61	54	48	43	40	37	35	33	32	30
0.55	1111	349	191	129	98	80	68	60	54	49	45	42	40	38	36	35
0.60	1171	374	207	142	109	89	76	67	61	56	52	49	46	44	42	40
0.70	1397	461	262	183	143	119	103	92	83	77	72	68	65	62	60	58
0.80	1912	651	378	269	213	179	157	141	129	120	113	107	102	98	95	92
0.90	3541	1241	736	533	427	362	320	290	267	250	236	225	216	208	201	196

Table 10d: Sample Size for a Hypothesis Test of the Odds Ratio
(Level of significance: **5%**; Power: **90%**; Alternative hypothesis: **2-sided**)

Odds Ratio (OR)

P^*_2	1.25	1.50	1.75	2.00	2.25	2.50	2.75	3.00	3.25	3.50	3.75	4.00	4.25	4.50	4.75	5.00
0.01	35761	9375	4355	2554	1700	1225	932	738	602	503	428	370	324	287	257	231
0.02	18133	4771	2224	1308	873	631	482	383	313	262	224	194	170	151	135	122
0.03	12261	3237	1514	894	598	434	332	264	217	182	156	135	119	106	95	86
0.04	9327	2472	1160	687	461	335	257	205	169	142	122	106	94	83	75	68
0.05	7569	2013	948	563	379	276	213	170	140	118	102	89	79	70	63	57
0.10	4072	1102	527	318	217	161	125	101	85	72	63	55	49	45	40	37
0.15	2929	807	392	240	166	124	98	80	68	58	51	46	41	37	34	32
0.20	2379	666	329	204	143	108	86	71	61	53	47	42	38	35	32	30
0.25	2068	589	295	185	131	101	81	68	58	51	45	41	37	34	32	30
0.30	1881	544	276	176	126	97	79	67	58	51	46	42	38	35	33	31
0.35	1769	519	267	172	125	97	80	68	59	52	47	43	40	37	35	33
0.40	1707	509	265	173	127	100	82	70	62	55	50	46	43	40	38	36
0.45	1686	510	269	177	131	104	87	75	66	59	54	50	46	43	41	39
0.50	1699	522	279	185	138	111	93	80	71	64	59	55	51	48	46	43
0.55	1747	544	294	198	149	120	101	88	78	71	66	61	57	54	51	49
0.60	1834	579	317	215	163	132	112	98	88	80	74	69	65	62	59	56
0.70	2170	704	394	272	209	172	148	130	118	108	101	94	89	85	82	78
0.80	2948	982	560	393	307	255	221	197	179	166	155	146	139	133	128	123
0.90	5421	1851	1076	766	606	509	445	399	366	340	319	303	289	278	268	259

Table 10e: Sample Size for a Hypothesis Test of the Odds Ratio
(Level of significance: **5%**; Power: **80%**; Alternative hypothesis: **2-sided**)

Odds Ratio (**OR**)

P^*_2	1.25	1.50	1.75	2.00	2.25	2.50	2.75	3.00	3.25	3.50	3.75	4.00	4.25	4.50	4.75	5.00
0.01	26421	6858	3157	1836	1213	868	656	516	419	348	295	254	221	195	174	156
0.02	13400	3492	1614	942	624	448	340	269	219	182	155	134	117	103	92	83
0.03	9063	2371	1100	644	429	309	235	186	152	127	108	94	82	73	65	59
0.04	6896	1811	843	496	331	239	183	145	119	100	85	74	65	58	52	47
0.05	5598	1476	690	407	272	198	151	121	99	83	71	62	55	49	44	40
0.10	3016	810	386	231	157	116	90	73	61	52	45	39	35	32	29	26
0.15	2172	595	288	175	121	90	71	58	49	42	37	33	30	27	25	23
0.20	1766	492	242	150	105	79	63	52	44	39	34	31	28	26	24	22
0.25	1537	436	218	137	97	74	60	50	43	38	33	30	28	26	24	22
0.30	1400	404	205	130	94	72	59	50	43	38	34	31	28	26	25	23
0.35	1318	387	199	128	93	73	60	51	44	39	36	32	30	28	26	25
0.40	1273	380	198	129	95	75	62	53	46	42	38	35	32	30	29	27
0.45	1259	381	202	133	98	78	65	56	50	45	41	38	35	33	31	30
0.50	1270	391	209	139	104	84	70	61	54	49	45	42	39	37	35	33
0.55	1307	408	221	149	112	91	77	67	60	54	50	47	44	42	40	38
0.60	1373	435	239	162	123	100	85	75	67	61	57	53	50	48	45	44
0.70	1629	531	298	206	159	131	113	100	91	83	78	73	69	66	63	61
0.80	2216	742	425	300	235	196	170	152	138	128	120	113	108	103	99	96
0.90	4083	1403	820	586	465	392	343	309	283	264	248	236	225	216	209	203

Table 10f: Sample Size for a Hypothesis Test of the Odds Ratio
(Level of significance: **5%**; Power: **50%**; Alternative hypothesis: **2-sided**)

Odds Ratio (**OR**)

P^*_2	1.25	1.50	1.75	2.00	2.25	2.50	2.75	3.00	3.25	3.50	3.75	4.00	4.25	4.50	4.75	5.00
0.01	12480	3136	1401	792	510	356	263	202	161	131	109	92	79	68	60	53
0.02	6335	1600	718	408	264	185	138	106	85	70	58	49	43	37	33	29
0.03	4289	1089	491	281	182	129	96	75	60	49	41	35	31	27	24	21
0.04	3266	833	378	217	142	100	75	59	47	39	33	28	25	22	19	17
0.05	2654	680	310	179	117	84	63	49	40	33	28	24	21	19	17	15
0.10	1436	377	176	104	70	51	39	31	26	22	19	17	15	13	12	11
0.15	1038	279	133	80	55	41	32	26	22	19	16	15	13	12	11	10
0.20	848	233	113	70	49	37	29	24	20	18	16	14	13	12	11	10
0.25	741	208	103	65	46	35	28	24	20	18	16	14	13	12	11	11
0.30	677	194	98	62	45	35	28	24	21	18	17	15	14	13	12	12
0.35	640	187	96	62	45	35	29	25	22	19	18	16	15	14	13	13
0.40	620	185	97	63	47	37	31	26	23	21	19	18	17	16	15	14
0.45	615	187	99	66	49	39	33	29	25	23	21	20	18	17	16	16
0.50	623	193	104	70	52	42	36	31	28	25	23	22	21	19	19	18
0.55	643	202	111	75	57	46	40	35	31	29	26	25	23	22	21	20
0.60	678	217	120	82	63	52	44	39	35	33	30	28	27	26	25	24
0.70	809	267	152	106	83	69	60	53	48	45	42	40	38	36	35	34
0.80	1107	377	219	156	123	104	91	82	75	70	66	62	59	57	55	53
0.90	2050	718	426	309	247	210	185	168	155	145	137	130	125	121	117	113

Table 10g: Sample Size for a Hypothesis Test of the Odds Ratio
(Level of significance: **10%**; Power: **90%**; Alternative hypothesis: **2-sided**)

Odds Ratio (**OR**)

P^*_2	1.25	1.50	1.75	2.00	2.25	2.50	2.75	3.00	3.25	3.50	3.75	4.00	4.25	4.50	4.75	5.00
0.01	29293	7713	3598	2117	1414	1022	780	619	506	424	362	313	275	244	218	197
0.02	14852	3924	1836	1084	726	526	403	321	263	221	189	164	144	128	115	104
0.03	10041	2662	1250	740	497	361	277	221	182	153	131	114	101	90	81	73
0.04	7638	2032	957	568	383	279	215	172	142	119	103	89	79	71	64	58
0.05	6197	1655	782	466	315	230	177	142	117	99	85	75	66	59	53	49
0.10	3332	905	434	262	180	133	104	84	70	60	52	46	41	37	34	31
0.15	2396	661	322	198	137	103	81	66	56	48	42	38	34	31	28	26
0.20	1944	546	270	168	118	89	71	59	50	44	39	35	31	29	27	25
0.25	1690	482	241	152	108	83	67	56	48	42	37	34	31	28	26	25
0.30	1536	445	226	144	103	80	65	55	47	42	37	34	31	29	27	25
0.35	1443	424	218	141	102	80	65	55	48	43	39	35	33	30	28	27
0.40	1393	415	217	141	103	81	67	57	50	45	41	37	35	32	31	29
0.45	1374	416	220	144	107	85	71	61	53	48	44	40	38	35	33	32
0.50	1385	425	227	151	113	90	75	65	58	52	48	44	41	39	37	35
0.55	1423	443	239	161	121	97	82	71	64	58	53	49	46	44	41	40
0.60	1493	471	257	174	132	107	91	79	71	65	60	56	52	50	47	45
0.70	1765	572	319	220	169	139	119	105	95	87	81	76	72	68	66	63
0.80	2396	796	453	318	247	206	178	158	144	133	124	117	111	107	102	99
0.90	4402	1499	870	618	488	409	357	321	293	272	256	242	231	222	214	207

Table 10h: Sample Size for a Hypothesis Test of the Odds Ratio
(Level of significance: **10%**; Power: **80%**; Alternative hypothesis: **2-sided**)

Odds Ratio (**OR**)

P^*_2	1.25	1.50	1.75	2.00	2.25	2.50	2.75	3.00	3.25	3.50	3.75	4.00	4.25	4.50	4.75	5.00
0.01	20906	5448	2518	1469	973	699	530	418	340	283	240	207	181	160	142	128
0.02	10603	2774	1286	753	501	361	274	217	177	148	126	109	95	84	76	68
0.03	7170	1883	876	515	344	248	189	150	123	103	88	76	67	59	53	48
0.04	5455	1438	672	396	265	192	147	117	96	81	69	60	53	47	42	38
0.05	4428	1172	549	325	218	159	122	97	80	67	58	50	44	40	36	32
0.10	2384	643	307	184	126	93	72	58	49	42	36	32	28	26	23	21
0.15	1716	471	228	140	97	72	57	47	39	34	30	26	24	22	20	18
0.20	1395	390	192	119	83	63	50	42	35	31	27	25	22	20	19	18
0.25	1214	345	173	108	77	59	47	40	34	30	27	24	22	20	19	18
0.30	1105	319	162	103	74	57	47	39	34	30	27	25	23	21	20	18
0.35	1039	305	157	101	73	57	47	40	35	31	28	26	24	22	21	20
0.40	1004	299	156	102	75	59	49	42	37	33	30	27	25	24	22	21
0.45	992	300	159	105	78	62	51	44	39	35	32	30	28	26	25	23
0.50	1000	308	165	110	82	66	55	48	42	38	35	33	31	29	27	26
0.55	1029	321	174	117	88	71	60	53	47	43	39	37	34	32	31	30
0.60	1081	342	188	127	97	79	67	59	53	48	44	42	39	37	35	34
0.70	1281	417	234	162	125	103	88	78	71	65	60	57	54	51	49	47
0.80	1742	582	333	234	183	153	132	118	108	100	93	88	84	80	77	75
0.90	3206	1099	641	458	362	305	267	240	220	205	193	183	175	168	162	157

Table 10i: Sample Size for a Hypothesis Test of the Odds Ratio
(Level of significance: **10%**;   Power: **50%**;   Alternative hypothesis: **2-sided**)

Odds Ratio (**OR**)

P^*_2	1.25	1.50	1.75	2.00	2.25	2.50	2.75	3.00	3.25	3.50	3.75	4.00	4.25	4.50	4.75	5.00
0.01	8791	2209	987	558	359	251	185	143	113	92	77	65	56	48	42	37
0.02	4463	1127	506	288	186	131	97	75	60	49	41	35	30	26	23	21
0.03	3021	767	346	198	129	91	68	53	42	35	29	25	22	19	17	15
0.04	2301	587	266	153	100	71	53	42	34	28	23	20	18	15	14	12
0.05	1869	479	219	126	83	59	44	35	28	24	20	17	15	13	12	11
0.10	1011	266	124	73	49	36	28	22	18	16	13	12	10	9	9	8
0.15	732	197	94	57	39	29	23	18	15	13	12	10	9	9	8	7
0.20	597	164	80	49	34	26	21	17	15	13	11	10	9	8	8	7
0.25	522	147	73	46	32	25	20	17	14	13	11	10	9	9	8	8
0.30	477	137	69	44	32	25	20	17	15	13	12	11	10	9	9	8
0.35	451	132	68	44	32	25	21	18	16	14	13	12	11	10	10	9
0.40	437	130	68	45	33	26	22	19	17	15	14	13	12	11	11	10
0.45	434	132	70	46	35	28	23	20	18	16	15	14	13	12	12	11
0.50	439	136	73	49	37	30	25	22	20	18	17	16	15	14	13	13
0.55	453	143	78	53	40	33	28	25	22	20	19	18	17	16	15	14
0.60	478	153	85	58	45	37	31	28	25	23	21	20	19	18	17	17
0.70	570	188	107	75	58	49	42	38	34	32	30	28	27	26	25	24
0.80	780	266	154	110	87	73	64	58	53	49	46	44	42	40	39	38
0.90	1444	506	300	218	174	148	131	118	109	102	97	92	88	85	82	80

Table 11a: Sample Size to Estimate the Relative Risk to Within 10 % of True Risk with **99%** Confidence

Relative Risk (**RR** ≤ 1/P₂)

P*₂	1.00	1.25	1.50	1.75	2.00	2.25	2.50	2.75	3.00	3.25	3.50	3.75	4.00	4.25	4.50	4.75	5.00
0.01	118359	106404	98434	92741	88471	85150	82493	80319	78508	76975	75661	74523	73527	72647	71866	71167	70538
0.02	58582	52604	48619	45773	43638	41977	40649	39562	38656	37890	37233	36664	36166	35726	35335	34986	34671
0.03	38656	34671	32015	30117	28694	27587	26701	25976	25373	24862	24424	24044	23712	23419	23159	22926	22716
0.04	28694	25705	23712	22289	21221	20391	19727	19184	18731	18348	18019	17734	17485	17266	17070	16895	16738
0.05	22716	20325	18731	17592	16738	16074	15543	15108	14746	14439	14176	13949	13749	13573	13417	13277	13151
0.10	10760	9565	8768	8199	7772	7439	7174	6956	6775	6622	6491	6377	6277	6189	6111	6041	5978
0.15	6775	5978	5447	5067	4783	4561	4384	4239	4118	4016	3929	3853	3786	3728	3676	3629	3587
0.20	4783	4185	3786	3502	3288	3122	2989	2881	2790	2713	2648	2591	2541	2497	2458	2423	2392
0.25	3587	3109	2790	2562	2392	2259	2152	2066	1993	1932	1879	1834	1794				
0.30	2790	2392	2126	1936	1794	1683	1595	1522		1411							
0.35	2221	1879	1651	1489	1367	1272	1196	1134									
0.40	1794	1495	1296	1153	1047	964	897										
0.45	1462	1196	1019	892	798												
0.50	1196	957	798	684	598												
0.55	979	761	616	513													
0.60	798	598	465														
0.70	513	342															
0.80	299	150															
0.90	133																

Table 11b: Sample Size to Estimate the Relative Risk to Within 20% of True Risk with **99%** Confidence

Relative Risk ($RR \leq 1/P_2$)

P^*_2	1.00	1.25	1.50	1.75	2.00	2.25	2.50	2.75	3.00	3.25	3.50	3.75	4.00	4.25	4.50	4.75	5.00
0.01	26387	23722	21945	20676	19724	18984	18391	17907	17503	17161	16868	16614	16392	16196	16022	15866	15726
0.02	13061	11728	10840	10205	9729	9359	9063	8820	8618	8448	8301	8174	8063	7965	7878	7800	7730
0.03	8618	7730	7138	6715	6397	6151	5953	5792	5657	5543	5445	5361	5287	5221	5163	5111	5065
0.04	6397	5731	5287	4969	4731	4546	4398	4277	4176	4091	4018	3954	3899	3850	3806	3767	3732
0.05	5065	4532	4176	3922	3732	3584	3465	3369	3288	3219	3161	3110	3066	3026	2992	2960	2932
0.10	2399	2133	1955	1828	1733	1659	1600	1551	1511	1477	1447	1422	1400	1380	1363	1347	1333
0.15	1511	1333	1215	1130	1067	1017	978	945	919	896	876	859	845	831	820	809	800
0.20	1067	933	845	781	733	696	667	643	622	605	591	578	567	557	548	541	534
0.25	800	693	622	572	534	504	480	461	445	431	419	409	400				
0.30	622	534	474	432	400	376	356	340	326	315							
0.35	495	419	369	332	305	284	267	253									
0.40	400	334	289	258	234	215	200										
0.45	326	267	228	199	178												
0.50	267	214	178	153	134												
0.55	219	170	138	115													
0.60	178	134	104														
0.70	115	77															
0.80	67	34															
0.90	30																

Table 11c: Sample Size to Estimate the Relative Risk to Within **25 %** of True Risk with **99%** Confidence

Relative Risk ($RR \leq 1/P_2$)

P_2^*	1.00	1.25	1.50	1.75	2.00	2.25	2.50	2.75	3.00	3.25	3.50	3.75	4.00	4.25	4.50	4.75	5.00
0.01	15876	14273	13203	12440	11867	11422	11065	10774	10531	10325	10149	9996	9863	9745	9640	9546	9462
0.02	7858	7056	6522	6140	5854	5631	5453	5307	5185	5083	4995	4918	4851	4792	4740	4693	4651
0.03	5185	4651	4295	4040	3849	3701	3582	3485	3404	3335	3276	3226	3181	3142	3107	3075	3047
0.04	3849	3448	3181	2990	2847	2736	2646	2574	2513	2461	2417	2379	2346	2316	2290	2267	2246
0.05	3047	2727	2513	2360	2246	2156	2085	2027	1978	1937	1902	1871	1845	1821	1800	1781	1764
0.10	1444	1283	1176	1100	1043	998	963	934	909	889	871	856	842	831	820	811	802
0.15	909	802	731	680	642	612	588	569	553	539	527	517	508	500	493	487	482
0.20	642	562	508	470	441	419	401	387	375	364	356	348	341	335	330	325	321
0.25	482	417	375	344	321	303	289	277	268	260	252	246	241				
0.30	375	321	286	260	241	226	214	205	196	190							
0.35	298	252	222	200	184	171	161	153									
0.40	241	201	174	155	141	130	121										
0.45	196	161	137	120	107												
0.50	161	129	107	92	81												
0.55	132	103	83	69													
0.60	107	81	63														
0.70	69	46															
0.80	41	21															
0.90	18																

Table 11d: Sample Size to Estimate the Relative Risk to Within
50 % of True Risk with 99% Confidence

Relative Risk ($RR \leq 1/P_2$)

P^*_2	1.00	1.25	1.50	1.75	2.00	2.25	2.50	2.75	3.00	3.25	3.50	3.75	4.00	4.25	4.50	4.75	5.00
0.01	2735	2459	2275	2143	2045	1968	1906	1856	1814	1779	1749	1722	1699	1679	1661	1645	1630
0.02	1354	1216	1124	1058	1009	970	940	915	894	876	861	848	836	826	817	809	802
0.03	894	802	740	696	663	638	617	601	587	575	565	556	548	542	536	530	525
0.04	663	594	548	515	491	472	456	444	433	424	417	410	404	399	395	391	387
0.05	525	470	433	407	387	372	360	350	341	334	328	323	318	314	310	307	304
0.10	249	221	203	190	180	172	166	161	157	153	150	148	146	143	142	140	139
0.15	157	139	126	118	111	106	102	98	96	93	91	90	88	87	85	84	83
0.20	111	97	88	81	76	73	70	67	65	63	62	60	59	58	57	56	56
0.25	83	72	65	60	56	53	50	48	47	45	44	43	42				
0.30	65	56	50	45	42	39	37	36	34	33							
0.35	52	44	39	35	32	30	28	27									
0.40	42	35	30	27	25	23	21										
0.45	34	28	24	21	19												
0.50	28	23	19	16	14												
0.55	23	18	15	12													
0.60	19	14	11														
0.70	12	8															
0.80	7	*															
0.90	*																

* Sample size less than 5

Table 11e: Sample Size to Estimate the Relative Risk to Within 10 % of True Risk with **95%** Confidence

Relative Risk ($RR \leq 1/P_2$)

P^*_2	1.00	1.25	1.50	1.75	2.00	2.25	2.50	2.75	3.00	3.25	3.50	3.75	4.00	4.25	4.50	4.75	5.00
0.01	68521	61600	56986	53690	51218	49295	47757	46499	45450	44563	43802	43143	42566	42057	41605	41200	40836
0.02	33915	30454	28147	26499	25263	24302	23533	22904	22379	21936	21555	21226	20937	20683	20457	20254	20072
0.03	22379	20072	18534	17436	16612	15971	15458	15039	14689	14393	14140	13920	13728	13558	13407	13272	13151
0.04	16612	14881	13728	12904	12286	11805	11421	11106	10844	10622	10432	10267	10123	9996	9883	9781	9690
0.05	13151	11767	10844	10185	9690	9306	8998	8746	8537	8359	8207	8075	7960	7858	7768	7687	7614
0.10	6230	5538	5076	4747	4499	4307	4153	4027	3923	3834	3758	3692	3634	3583	3538	3498	3461
0.15	3923	3461	3154	2934	2769	2641	2538	2454	2384	2325	2275	2231	2192	2158	2128	2101	2077
0.20	2769	2423	2192	2027	1904	1808	1731	1668	1615	1571	1533	1500	1471	1446	1423	1403	1385
0.25	2077	1800	1615	1484	1385	1308	1246	1196	1154	1119	1088	1062	1039				
0.30	1615	1385	1231	1121	1039	975	923	881		817							
0.35	1286	1088	956	862	792	737	693	657									
0.40	1039	866	750	668	606	558	520										
0.45	846	693	590	517	462												
0.50	693	554	462	396	347												
0.55	567	441	357	297													
0.60	462	347	270														
0.70	297	198															
0.80	174	87															
0.90	77																

Table 11f: Sample Size to Estimate the Relative Risk to Within 20 % of True Risk with **95%** Confidence

Relative Risk ($RR \leq 1/P_2$)

P^*_2	1.00	1.25	1.50	1.75	2.00	2.25	2.50	2.75	3.00	3.25	3.50	3.75	4.00	4.25	4.50	4.75	5.00
0.01	15276	13733	12705	11970	11419	10990	10647	10367	10133	9935	9766	9619	9490	9377	9276	9186	9104
0.02	7561	6790	6275	5908	5633	5418	5247	5107	4990	4891	4806	4732	4668	4611	4561	4516	4475
0.03	4990	4475	4132	3887	3704	3561	3447	3353	3275	3209	3153	3104	3061	3023	2989	2959	2932
0.04	3704	3318	3061	2877	2739	2632	2546	2476	2418	2368	2326	2289	2257	2229	2204	2181	2161
0.05	2932	2624	2418	2271	2161	2075	2006	1950	1904	1864	1830	1801	1775	1752	1732	1714	1698
0.10	1389	1235	1132	1059	1003	961	926	898	875	855	838	823	811	799	789	780	772
0.15	875	772	703	654	618	589	566	548	532	519	507	498	489	482	475	469	463
0.20	618	541	489	452	425	403	386	372	361	351	342	335	328	323	318	313	309
0.25	463	402	361	331	309	292	278	267	258	250	243	237	232				
0.30	361	309	275	250	232	218	206	197	189	182							
0.35	287	243	214	193	177	165	155	147									
0.40	232	193	168	149	136	125	116										
0.45	189	155	132	116	103												
0.50	155	124	103	89	78												
0.55	127	99	80	67													
0.60	103	78	61														
0.70	67	45															
0.80	39	20															
0.90	18																

Table 11g: Sample Size to Estimate the Relative Risk to Within 25 % of True Risk with **95%** Confidence

Relative Risk (**RR** ≤ 1/**P**$_2$)

P*$_2$	1.00	1.25	1.50	1.75	2.00	2.25	2.50	2.75	3.00	3.25	3.50	3.75	4.00	4.25	4.50	4.75	5.00
0.01	9191	8263	7644	7202	6870	6612	6406	6237	6097	5978	5876	5787	5710	5642	5581	5527	5478
0.02	4549	4085	3776	3555	3389	3260	3157	3073	3002	2943	2892	2847	2809	2775	2744	2717	2693
0.03	3002	2693	2486	2339	2229	2143	2074	2018	1971	1931	1897	1868	1842	1819	1799	1781	1764
0.04	2229	1996	1842	1731	1648	1584	1532	1490	1455	1425	1400	1378	1358	1341	1326	1312	1300
0.05	1764	1579	1455	1367	1300	1249	1207	1174	1145	1122	1101	1084	1068	1054	1042	1031	1022
0.10	836	743	681	637	604	578	558	541	527	515	504	496	488	481	475	470	465
0.15	527	465	423	394	372	355	341	330	320	312	306	300	294	290	286	282	279
0.20	372	325	294	272	256	243	233	224	217	211	206	202	198	194	191	189	186
0.25	279	242	217	199	186	176	168	161	155	150	146	143	140				
0.30	217	186	166	151	140	131	124	119	114	110							
0.35	173	146	129	116	107	99	93	89									
0.40	140	117	101	90	82	75	70										
0.45	114	93	80	70	62												
0.50	93	75	62	54	47												
0.55	76	60	48	40													
0.60	62	47	37														
0.70	40	27															
0.80	24	12															
0.90	11																

Table 11h: Sample Size to Estimate the Relative Risk to Within 50 % of True Risk with **95%** Confidence

Relative Risk (**RR** ≤ 1/P₂)

P*₂	1.00	1.25	1.50	1.75	2.00	2.25	2.50	2.75	3.00	3.25	3.50	3.75	4.00	4.25	4.50	4.75	5.00
0.01	1584	1424	1317	1241	1184	1139	1104	1075	1051	1030	1013	997	984	972	962	952	944
0.02	784	704	651	613	584	562	544	530	518	507	499	491	484	478	473	468	464
0.03	518	464	429	403	384	369	358	348	340	333	327	322	318	314	310	307	304
0.04	384	344	318	299	284	273	264	257	251	246	242	238	234	231	229	226	224
0.05	304	272	251	236	224	215	208	203	198	194	190	187	184	182	180	178	176
0.10	144	128	118	110	104	100	96	94	91	89	87	86	84	83	82	81	80
0.15	91	80	73	68	64	62	59	57	56	54	53	52	51	50	50	49	48
0.20	64	56	51	47	44	42	40	39	38	37	36	35	34	34	33	33	32
0.25	48	42	38	35	32	31	29	28	27	26	26	25	24				
0.30	38	32	29	26	24	23	22	21	20	19							
0.35	30	26	23	20	19	18	16	16									
0.40	24	20	18	16	14	13	12										
0.45	20	16	14	12	11												
0.50	16	13	11	10	8												
0.55	14	11	9	7													
0.60	11	8	7														
0.70	7	5															
0.80	*	*															
0.90	*																

* Sample size less than 5

Table 11i: Sample Size to Estimate the Relative Risk to Within 10 % of True Risk with 90% Confidence

Relative Risk ($RR \le 1/P_2$)

P^{*}_2	1.00	1.25	1.50	1.75	2.00	2.25	2.50	2.75	3.00	3.25	3.50	3.75	4.00	4.25	4.50	4.75	5.00
0.01	48266	43391	40141	37819	36078	34724	33640	32754	32015	31390	30855	30390	29984	29625	29307	29022	28765
0.02	23890	21452	19827	18666	17796	17118	16577	16133	15764	15452	15184	14952	14748	14569	14410	14267	14139
0.03	15764	14139	13056	12282	11701	11250	10889	10593	10347	10139	9960	9805	9670	9550	9444	9349	9264
0.04	11701	10483	9670	9090	8654	8316	8045	7823	7639	7482	7348	7232	7131	7041	6961	6890	6826
0.05	9264	8289	7639	7174	6826	6555	6338	6161	6013	5888	5781	5688	5607	5535	5472	5415	5363
0.10	4388	3901	3576	3344	3169	3034	2926	2837	2763	2701	2647	2601	2560	2524	2492	2464	2438
0.15	2763	2438	2221	2067	1951	1860	1788	1729	1680	1638	1602	1571	1544	1520	1499	1480	1463
0.20	1951	1707	1544	1428	1341	1274	1219	1175	1138	1107	1080	1057	1037	1019	1003	988	976
0.25	1463	1268	1138	1045	976	921	878	843	813	788	767	748	732				
0.30	1138	976	867	790	732	687	651	621		576							
0.35	906	767	674	607	558	519	488	463									
0.40	732	610	529	471	427	393	366										
0.45	596	488	416	364	326												
0.50	488	391	326	279	244												
0.55	399	311	252	209													
0.60	326	244	190														
0.70	209	140															
0.80	122	61															
0.90	55																

Table 11j: Sample Size to Estimate the Relative Risk to Within 20 % of True Risk with **90%** Confidence

Relative Risk (**RR** $\leq$ 1/P$_2$)

P*$_2$	1.00	1.25	1.50	1.75	2.00	2.25	2.50	2.75	3.00	3.25	3.50	3.75	4.00	4.25	4.50	4.75	5.00
0.01	10761	9674	8949	8432	8044	7742	7500	7303	7138	6999	6879	6776	6685	6605	6534	6470	6413
0.02	5326	4783	4421	4162	3968	3817	3696	3597	3515	3445	3385	3334	3288	3248	3213	3181	3153
0.03	3515	3153	2911	2738	2609	2508	2428	2362	2307	2261	2221	2186	2156	2130	2106	2085	2066
0.04	2609	2337	2156	2027	1930	1854	1794	1744	1703	1668	1639	1613	1590	1570	1552	1536	1522
0.05	2066	1848	1703	1600	1522	1462	1413	1374	1341	1313	1289	1269	1250	1234	1220	1208	1196
0.10	979	870	798	746	707	677	653	633	616	602	591	580	571	563	556	550	544
0.15	616	544	496	461	435	415	399	386	375	366	358	351	345	339	335	330	327
0.20	435	381	345	319	299	284	272	262	254	247	241	236	231	227	224	221	218
0.25	327	283	254	233	218	206	196	188	182	176	171	167	164				
0.30	254	218	194	176	164	153	145	139	133	129							
0.35	202	171	151	136	125	116	109	104									
0.40	164	136	118	105	96	88	82										
0.45	133	109	93	82	73												
0.50	109	87	73	63	55												
0.55	89	70	56	47													
0.60	73	55	43														
0.70	47	32															
0.80	28	14															
0.90	13																

Table 11k: Sample Size to Estimate the Relative Risk to Within **25 %** of True Risk with **90%** Confidence

Relative Risk (RR ≤ 1/P_2)

P^*_2	1.00	1.25	1.50	1.75	2.00	2.25	2.50	2.75	3.00	3.25	3.50	3.75	4.00	4.25	4.50	4.75	5.00
0.01	6474	5821	5385	5073	4840	4658	4513	4394	4295	4211	4139	4077	4022	3974	3931	3893	3859
0.02	3205	2878	2660	2504	2387	2297	2224	2164	2115	2073	2037	2006	1979	1955	1933	1914	1897
0.03	2115	1897	1752	1648	1570	1509	1461	1421	1388	1360	1336	1316	1297	1281	1267	1254	1243
0.04	1570	1406	1297	1220	1161	1116	1079	1050	1025	1004	986	971	957	945	934	925	916
0.05	1243	1112	1025	963	916	880	851	827	807	790	776	763	753	743	734	727	720
0.10	589	524	480	449	426	407	393	381	371	363	355	349	344	339	335	331	327
0.15	371	327	298	278	262	250	240	232	226	220	215	211	208	204	202	199	197
0.20	262	229	208	192	180	171	164	158	153	149	145	142	139	137	135	133	131
0.25	197	171	153	141	131	124	118	113	109	106	103	101	99				
0.30	153	131	117	106	99	93	88	84	80	78							
0.35	122	103	91	82	75	70	66	62									
0.40	99	82	71	64	58	53	50										
0.45	80	66	56	49	44												
0.50	66	53	44	38	33												
0.55	54	42	34	29													
0.60	44	33	26														
0.70	29	19															
0.80	17	9															
0.90	8																

Table 11I: Sample Size to Estimate the Relative Risk to Within 50 % of True Risk with 90% Confidence

Relative Risk (RR ≤ 1/P₂)

P*₂	1.00	1.25	1.50	1.75	2.00	2.25	2.50	2.75	3.00	3.25	3.50	3.75	4.00	4.25	4.50	4.75	5.00
0.01	1116	1003	928	874	834	803	778	757	740	726	713	703	693	685	678	671	665
0.02	552	496	459	432	412	396	383	373	365	357	351	346	341	337	333	330	327
0.03	365	327	302	284	271	260	252	245	240	235	231	227	224	221	219	217	215
0.04	271	243	224	211	200	193	186	181	177	173	170	168	165	163	161	160	158
0.05	215	192	177	166	158	152	147	143	139	137	134	132	130	128	127	126	124
0.10	102	91	83	78	74	71	68	66	64	63	62	61	60	59	58	57	57
0.15	64	57	52	48	46	43	42	40	39	38	38	37	36	36	35	35	34
0.20	46	40	36	33	31	30	29	28	27	26	25	25	24	24	24	23	23
0.25	34	30	27	25	23	22	21	20	19	19	18	18	17				
0.30	27	23	21	19	17	16	16	15	14	14							
0.35	21	18	16	15	13	12	12	11									
0.40	17	15	13	11	10	10	9										
0.45	14	12	10	9	8												
0.50	12	10	8	7	6												
0.55	10	8	6	5													
0.60	8	6	5														
0.70	5	*															
0.80	*	*															
0.90	*																

* Sample size less than 5

Table 12a: Sample Size for a Hypothesis Test of the Relative Risk
(Level of significance:1%; Power: **90%**; Alternative hypothesis: **2-sided**)

Relative Risk (**RR** $\leq$ **1/P₂**)

P^*_2	1.00	1.25	1.50	1.75	2.00	2.25	2.50	2.75	3.00	3.25	3.50	3.75	4.00	4.25	4.50	4.75	5.00
0.01	52978	14696	7175	4396	3044	2273	1786	1457	1221	1046	911	804	718	648	589	539	
0.02	26187	7254	3536	2164	1496	1115	875	712	596	510	443	391	349	314	285	260	
0.03	17256	4773	2324	1419	980	729	571	464	388	331	287	253	225	202	183	167	
0.04	12791	3533	1717	1047	722	536	419	340	284	242	210	184	164	147	133	121	
0.05	10112	2789	1353	824	567	421	328	266	221	188	163	143	127	113	102	93	
0.10	4754	1300	626	378	257	189	146	117	96	81	69	60	53	46	41	37	
0.15	2967	804	383	229	154	112	85	67	55	45	38	32	28	24	21	18	
0.20	2074	556	262	154	102	73	55	43	34	27	22	19	15	13	11	9	
0.25	1539	407	189	110	72	50	37	28	21	17	13	10					
0.30	1181	308	141	80	51	35	24	18	13								
0.35	926	237	106	59	36	24	16										
0.40	735	184	80	43	25	15											
0.45	586	143	60	30													
0.50	467	110	43	20													
0.55	369	83	30														
0.60	288	60															
0.70	161																
0.80	65																

Table 12b: Sample Size for a Hypothesis Test of the Relative Risk

(Level of significance: 1%; Power: **80%**; Alternative hypothesis: **2-sided**)

Relative Risk (**RR** $\leq 1/P_2$)

P^*_2	1.00	1.25	1.50	1.75	2.00	2.25	2.50	2.75	3.00	3.25	3.50	3.75	4.00	4.25	4.50	4.75	5.00
0.01	41584	11536	5632	3451	2390	1785	1403	1144	959	821	715	632	564	509	463	424	
0.02	20555	5694	2776	1699	1175	876	688	560	469	401	349	307	274	247	224	205	
0.03	13545	3747	1824	1115	770	573	449	365	305	261	226	199	177	159	145	132	
0.04	10040	2774	1348	823	567	422	330	268	223	190	165	145	129	116	105	95	
0.05	7937	2190	1063	647	446	331	258	209	174	148	128	113	100	90	81	74	
0.10	3732	1021	492	297	203	149	115	93	76	64	55	48	42	37	33	30	
0.15	2330	632	301	180	122	88	68	54	44	36	30	26	22	20	17	15	
0.20	1629	437	206	122	81	58	44	34	27	22	18	15	13	11	9	8	
0.25	1208	320	149	87	57	40	29	22	17	14	11	9					
0.30	928	242	111	63	41	28	20	15	11								
0.35	728	187	84	47	29	19	13										
0.40	577	145	63	34	20	13											
0.45	461	113	47	24													
0.50	367	87	35	16													
0.55	291	65	24														
0.60	227	48															
0.70	127																
0.80	52																

Table 12c: Sample Size for a Hypothesis Test of the Relative Risk
(Level of significance:1%; Power: **50%**; Alternative hypothesis: **2-sided**)

Relative Risk (**RR** $\leq$ 1/P_2)

P^*_2	1.00	1.25	1.50	1.75	2.00	2.25	2.50	2.75	3.00	3.25	3.50	3.75	4.00	4.25	4.50	4.75	5.00
0.01	23621	6553	3200	1961	1358	1015	798	651	546	468	407	360	322	290	264	242	
0.02	11676	3235	1578	966	668	499	392	319	267	229	199	176	157	141	128	117	
0.03	7695	2129	1037	634	438	327	256	208	174	149	130	114	102	92	83	76	
0.04	5704	1576	767	468	323	240	188	153	128	109	95	83	74	67	61	55	
0.05	4510	1245	605	369	254	189	148	120	100	85	74	65	58	52	47	43	
0.10	2121	581	280	170	116	86	67	54	44	38	32	28	25	22	20	18	
0.15	1324	360	172	103	70	51	39	31	26	22	18	16	14	12	11	10	
0.20	926	249	118	70	47	34	26	20	17	14	11	10	8	7	6	5	
0.25	687	183	86	50	33	24	18	14	11	9	7	6					
0.30	528	139	64	37	24	17	12	9	7								
0.35	414	107	49	28	18	12	8										
0.40	329	83	37	20	13	8											
0.45	263	65	28	15													
0.50	210	50	21	10													
0.55	166	38	15														
0.60	130	28															
0.70	73																
0.80	30																

Table 12d: Sample Size for a Hypothesis Test of the Relative Risk
(Level of significance:**5%**; Power: **90%**; Alternative hypothesis: **2-sided**)

Relative Risk ($RR \le 1/P_2$)

P^*_2	1.00	1.25	1.50	1.75	2.00	2.25	2.50	2.75	3.00	3.25	3.50	3.75	4.00	4.25	4.50	4.75	5.00
0.01	37411	10378	5066	3104	2149	1605	1261	1028	862	738	643	568	507	457	416	381	
0.02	18492	5122	2497	1528	1056	787	618	503	421	360	313	276	246	221	201	184	
0.03	12185	3371	1641	1002	692	515	403	328	274	234	203	178	159	143	129	118	
0.04	9032	2495	1212	739	509	379	296	240	200	171	148	130	115	103	93	85	
0.05	7140	1969	955	582	400	297	232	188	156	133	115	101	89	80	72	65	
0.10	3357	918	442	266	182	133	103	82	68	57	49	42	37	33	29	26	
0.15	2095	568	270	161	109	79	60	47	38	32	27	23	19	17	15	13	
0.20	1465	393	185	109	72	52	39	30	24	19	16	13	11	9	7	6	
0.25	1086	287	133	77	50	35	26	19	15	12	9	7					
0.30	834	217	99	56	36	24	17	12	9								
0.35	654	167	75	41	25	16	11										
0.40	519	130	56	30	17	11											
0.45	414	101	42	21													
0.50	329	77	30	14													
0.55	261	58	21														
0.60	203	42															
0.70	113																
0.80	46																

Table 12e: Sample Size for a Hypothesis Test of the Relative Risk
(Level of significance:**5%**; Power: **80%**; Alternative hypothesis: **2-sided**)

Relative Risk ($RR \leq 1/P_2$)

P_2^*	1.00	1.25	1.50	1.75	2.00	2.25	2.50	2.75	3.00	3.25	3.50	3.75	4.00	4.25	4.50	4.75	5.00
0.01	27946	7752	3785	2319	1606	1199	943	769	644	552	481	425	379	342	311	285	
0.02	13814	3827	1866	1142	789	589	462	376	315	269	234	207	184	166	151	138	
0.03	9103	2518	1226	749	517	385	302	245	205	175	152	134	119	107	97	89	
0.04	6747	1864	906	553	381	283	222	180	150	128	111	97	87	78	70	64	
0.05	5334	1471	714	435	299	222	174	141	117	100	86	76	67	60	54	49	
0.10	2508	686	330	200	136	100	77	62	51	43	37	32	28	25	22	20	
0.15	1566	425	202	121	82	59	45	36	29	24	20	17	15	13	11	10	
0.20	1095	294	138	82	54	39	29	23	18	15	12	10	8	7	6	5	
0.25	812	215	100	58	38	27	20	15	12	9	7	6					
0.30	623	163	74	42	27	19	13	10	7								
0.35	489	125	56	31	19	13	9										
0.40	388	97	42	23	14	8											
0.45	309	76	32	16													
0.50	247	58	23	11													
0.55	195	44	16														
0.60	152	32															
0.70	85																
0.80	35																

Table 12f: Sample Size for a Hypothesis Test of the Relative Risk
(Level of significance:**5%**; Power: **50%**; Alternative hypothesis: **2-sided**)

Relative Risk (RR $\leq 1/P_2$)

P^*_2	1.00	1.25	1.50	1.75	2.00	2.25	2.50	2.75	3.00	3.25	3.50	3.75	4.00	4.25	4.50	4.75	5.00
0.01	13675	3794	1853	1136	787	588	462	377	316	271	236	209	186	168	153	140	
0.02	6760	1873	914	559	387	289	227	185	155	133	115	102	91	82	75	68	
0.03	4455	1233	601	367	254	189	148	121	101	86	75	66	59	53	48	44	
0.04	3302	913	444	271	187	139	109	89	74	63	55	49	43	39	35	32	
0.05	2611	721	350	214	147	110	86	70	58	50	43	38	34	30	27	25	
0.10	1228	337	162	98	67	50	39	31	26	22	19	17	15	13	12	11	
0.15	767	209	100	60	41	30	23	18	15	13	11	9	8	7	6	6	
0.20	536	145	69	41	27	20	15	12	10	8	7	6	5	*	*	*	
0.25	398	106	50	29	19	14	10	8	7	5	*	*					
0.30	306	81	37	22	14	10	7	6	*								
0.35	240	62	28	16	10	7	5										
0.40	191	49	22	12	10	7	5										
0.45	152	38	16	9	7	5											
0.50	122	29	12	6													
0.55	96	22	9														
0.60	75	17															
0.70	42																
0.80	18																

*Sample size less than 5

Table 12g: Sample Size for a Hypothesis Test of the Relative Risk
(Level of significance: **10%**; Power: **90%**; Alternative hypothesis: **2-sided**)

Relative Risk (RR $\leq$ 1/P_2)

P_2^*	1.00	1.25	1.50	1.75	2.00	2.25	2.50	2.75	3.00	3.25	3.50	3.75	4.00	4.25	4.50	4.75	5.00
0.01	30494	8459	4130	2530	1752	1308	1028	838	703	602	524	463	413	373	339	310	
0.02	15073	4175	2035	1245	861	642	503	410	343	293	255	225	200	180	164	150	
0.03	9932	2747	1337	817	564	420	329	267	223	190	165	145	129	116	105	96	
0.04	7362	2033	988	603	415	308	241	196	163	139	120	106	94	84	76	69	
0.05	5820	1605	779	474	326	242	189	153	127	108	93	82	73	65	59	53	
0.10	2736	748	360	217	148	109	84	67	55	46	40	34	30	26	24	21	
0.15	1708	463	220	131	88	64	49	39	31	26	22	18	16	14	12	10	
0.20	1194	320	150	89	59	42	31	24	19	16	13	10	9	7	6	5	
0.25	885	234	109	63	41	29	21	16	12	9	7	6					
0.30	680	177	81	46	29	20	14	10	7								
0.35	533	136	61	33	21	13	9										
0.40	423	106	46	24	14	8											
0.45	337	82	34	17													
0.50	268	63	25	11													
0.55	212	47	17														
0.60	166	34															
0.70	92																
0.80	37																

Table 12h: Sample Size for a Hypothesis Test of the Relative Risk
(Level of significance: **10%**; Power: **80%**; Alternative hypothesis: **2-sided**)

Relative Risk ($RR \leq 1/P_2$)

P_2^*	1.00	1.25	1.50	1.75	2.00	2.25	2.50	2.75	3.00	3.25	3.50	3.75	4.00	4.25	4.50	4.75	5.00
0.01	22016	6107	2982	1827	1265	945	743	606	508	435	379	334	299	270	245	224	
0.02	10882	3015	1470	899	622	464	364	296	248	212	184	163	145	131	119	108	
0.03	7171	1984	966	590	407	303	238	193	161	138	120	105	94	84	76	70	
0.04	5316	1468	714	436	300	223	175	142	118	101	87	77	68	61	55	50	
0.05	4202	1159	563	343	236	175	137	111	92	78	68	60	53	47	43	39	
0.10	1976	541	260	157	107	79	61	49	40	34	29	25	22	20	17	16	
0.15	1233	334	159	95	64	47	36	28	23	19	16	14	12	10	9	8	
0.20	862	231	109	64	43	31	23	18	14	12	10	8	7	6	5	*	
0.25	640	170	79	46	30	21	16	12	9	7	6	*					
0.30	491	128	59	33	21	15	10	8	6								
0.35	385	99	44	25	15	10	7										
0.40	306	77	33	18	11	7											
0.45	244	60	25	13													
0.50	194	46	18	9													
0.55	154	35	13														
0.60	120	25															
0.70	67																
0.80	27																

* Sample size less than 5

Table 12i: Sample Size for a Hypothesis Test of the Relative Risk
(Level of significance: **10%**; Power: **50%**; Alternative hypothesis: **2-sided**)

Relative Risk ($RR \leq 1/P_2$)

P_2^*	1.00	1.25	1.50	1.75	2.00	2.25	2.50	2.75	3.00	3.25	3.50	3.75	4.00	4.25	4.50	4.75	5.00
0.01	9633	2673	1305	800	554	414	326	266	223	191	166	147	131	119	108	99	
0.02	4762	1320	644	394	273	204	160	130	109	94	81	72	64	58	53	48	
0.03	3138	869	423	259	179	133	105	85	71	61	53	47	42	38	34	31	
0.04	2326	643	313	191	132	98	77	63	52	45	39	34	31	28	25	23	
0.05	1839	508	247	151	104	77	61	49	41	35	30	27	24	21	19	18	
0.10	865	237	115	70	48	35	27	22	18	16	13	12	10	9	8	8	
0.15	540	147	71	42	29	21	16	13	11	9	8	7	6	5	5	*	
0.20	378	102	48	29	19	14	11	9	7	6	5	*	*	*	*	*	
0.25	281	75	35	21	14	10	8	6	5	*	*	*					
0.30	216	57	26	15	10	7	5	*									
0.35	169	44	20	12	7	5	*										
0.40	134	34	15	9	5												
0.45	107	27	12	7	5	*											
0.50	86	21	9	5													
0.55	68	16	6														
0.60	53	12	6														
0.70	30																
0.80	13																

* Sample size less than 5

Table 13a: Sample Sizes for Lot Quality Assurance Sampling
No case acceptable with **99** % confidence

Prevalence %

Population	90	80	70	60	50	40	30	20	10	5	2.5	1.25
100	2	3	4	5	7	9	13	19	36	59	90	98
200	2	3	4	5	7	9	13	20	40	73	120	182
1000	2	3	4	6	7	9	13	21	43	86	167	307
2000	2	3	4	6	7	9	13	21	44	88	174	335
2500	2	3	4	6	7	9	13	21	44	89	176	341
5000	3	3	4	6	7	10	13	21	44	89	179	354
10000	3	3	4	6	7	10	13	21	44	90	181	360
15000	3	3	4	6	7	10	13	21	44	90	181	361
20000	3	3	4	6	7	10	13	21	44	90	182	364
25000	3	3	4	6	7	10	13	21	44	90	182	365
50000	3	3	4	6	7	10	14	21	45	91	182	365
Infinite	3	3	4	6	7	10	14	21	45	91	182	367

Table 13b: Sample Sizes for Lot Quality Assurance Sampling
No more than **1** case acceptable with **.99%** confidence

Prevalence %

Population	90	80	70	60	50	40	30	20	10	5	2.5	1.25
100	4	5	6	8	10	13	18	27	49	76	98	100
200	4	5	6	8	10	14	19	29	56	98	153	196
1000	4	5	7	8	11	14	19	30	62	123	234	422
2000	4	5	7	8	11	14	20	31	63	127	248	470
2500	4	5	7	8	11	14	20	31	63	128	252	483
5000	4	5	7	8	11	14	20	31	64	129	257	506
10000	4	5	7	8	11	14	20	31	64	129	260	516
15000	4	5	7	8	11	14	20	31	64	130	261	520
20000	4	5	7	8	11	14	20	31	64	130	261	525
25000	4	5	7	8	11	14	20	31	64	130	262	525
50000	4	5	7	8	11	14	20	31	65	131	263	526
Infinite	4	5	7	8	11	14	20	31	65	131	263	529

Table 13c: Sample Sizes for Lot Quality Assurance Sampling
No more than **2** cases acceptable with **99%** confidence

Prevalence %

Population	90	80	70	60	50	40	30	20	10	5	2.5	1.25
100	5	7	8	10	13	17	23	33	59	87	100	100
200	5	7	8	11	13	17	24	36	69	119	175	200
1000	5	7	9	11	14	18	25	39	79	155	291	516
2000	5	7	9	11	14	18	25	39	80	160	311	584
2500	5	7	9	11	14	18	25	39	80	161	317	604
5000	5	7	9	11	14	18	25	39	81	163	326	637
10000	5	7	9	11	14	18	25	39	81	164	329	653
15000	5	7	9	11	14	18	25	39	81	164	329	658
20000	5	7	9	11	14	18	25	39	81	165	332	665
25000	5	7	9	11	14	18	25	39	81	165	333	666
50000	5	7	9	11	14	18	25	39	82	166	333	668
Infinite	5	7	9	11	14	18	25	39	82	166	334	670

Table 13d: Sample Sizes for Lot Quality Assurance Sampling
No more than **3** cases acceptable with **99%** confidence

Prevalence %

Population	90	80	70	60	50	40	30	20	10	5	2.5	1.25
100	7	8	10	13	16	20	27	39	67	95	100	100
200	7	8	10	13	16	21	29	43	81	136	190	200
1000	7	9	11	13	17	22	30	46	94	183	342	597
2000	7	9	11	13	17	22	30	47	96	191	369	687
2500	7	9	11	13	17	22	30	47	96	192	377	713
5000	7	9	11	13	17	22	30	47	97	195	388	757
10000	7	9	11	13	17	22	30	47	97	197	393	778
15000	7	9	11	13	17	22	30	47	97	197	394	785
20000	7	9	11	13	17	22	30	47	97	197	396	793
25000	7	9	11	13	17	22	30	47	97	198	397	794
50000	7	9	11	13	17	22	30	47	98	198	397	794
Infinite	7	9	11	13	17	22	30	47	98	198	399	801

Table 13e: Sample Sizes for Lot Quality Assurance Sampling
No more than **4** cases acceptable with **99%** confidence

Prevalence %

Population	90	80	70	60	50	40	30	20	10	5	2.5	1.25
100	8	10	12	15	18	23	31	45	75	100	100	100
200	8	10	12	15	19	24	33	49	92	151	199	200
1000	8	10	12	15	19	25	35	54	109	210	390	669
2000	8	10	12	15	19	25	35	54	111	220	424	781
2500	8	10	12	15	19	25	35	54	111	222	434	816
5000	8	10	12	15	19	25	35	54	112	225	447	871
10000	8	10	12	15	19	25	35	54	112	227	454	897
15000	8	10	12	15	19	25	35	55	112	227	455	906
20000	8	10	12	15	19	25	35	55	113	228	457	912
25000	8	10	12	15	19	25	35	55	113	228	460	917
50000	8	10	12	15	19	25	35	55	113	230	460	917
Infinite	8	10	12	15	19	25	35	55	113	230	461	925

Table 13f: Sample Sizes for Lot Quality Assurance Sampling
No case acceptable with **95%** confidence

Prevalence %

Population	90	80	70	60	50	40	30	20	10	5	2.5	1.25
100	2	2	3	4	5	6	9	13	25	45	82	96
200	2	2	3	4	5	6	9	13	27	51	90	140
1000	2	2	3	4	5	6	9	14	29	57	112	212
2000	2	2	3	4	5	6	9	14	29	58	115	225
2500	2	2	3	4	5	6	9	14	29	58	116	228
5000	2	2	3	4	5	6	9	14	29	58	118	234
10000	2	2	3	4	5	6	9	14	29	59	118	236
15000	2	2	3	4	5	6	9	14	29	59	118	237
20000	2	2	3	4	5	6	9	14	29	59	118	238
25000	2	2	3	4	5	6	9	14	29	59	119	238
50000	2	2	3	4	5	6	9	14	29	59	119	239
Infinite	2	2	3	4	5	6	9	14	29	59	119	239

Table 13g: Sample Sizes for Lot Quality Assurance Sampling
No more than **1** case acceptable with **95%** confidence

Prevalence %

Population	90	80	70	60	50	40	30	20	10	5	2.5	1.25
100	3	4	5	6	8	10	14	20	38	64	95	100
200	3	4	5	6	8	10	14	21	42	77	127	191
1000	3	4	5	6	8	10	14	22	45	90	174	324
2000	3	4	5	6	8	10	14	22	46	92	181	348
2500	3	4	5	6	8	10	14	22	46	92	183	356
5000	3	4	5	6	8	10	14	22	46	93	186	367
10000	3	4	5	6	8	10	14	22	46	93	187	372
15000	3	4	5	6	8	10	14	22	46	93	187	374
20000	3	4	5	6	8	10	14	22	46	93	188	376
25000	3	4	5	6	8	10	14	22	46	93	188	379
50000	3	4	5	6	8	10	14	22	46	94	188	379
Infinite	3	4	5	6	8	10	14	22	46	94	188	379

Table 13h: Sample Sizes for Lot Quality Assurance Sampling
No more than **2** cases acceptable with **95%** confidence

Prevalence %

Population	90	80	70	60	50	40	30	20	10	5	2.5	1.25
100	4	6	7	8	10	13	18	27	48	77	100	100
200	5	6	7	8	11	14	19	28	54	98	155	200
1000	5	6	7	8	11	14	19	29	60	118	227	417
2000	5	6	7	8	11	14	19	30	61	122	238	455
2500	5	6	7	8	11	14	19	30	61	122	242	467
5000	5	6	7	8	11	14	19	30	61	123	246	486
10000	5	6	7	9	11	14	19	30	61	123	248	493
15000	5	6	7	9	11	14	19	30	61	124	248	497
20000	5	6	7	9	11	14	19	30	61	124	251	502
25000	5	6	7	9	11	14	19	30	62	124	251	502
50000	5	6	7	9	11	14	19	30	62	125	251	502
Infinite	5	6	7	9	11	14	19	30	62	125	251	502

Table 13i: Sample Sizes for Lot Quality Assurance Sampling
No more than **3** cases acceptable with **95%** confidence

Prevalence %

Population	90	80	70	60	50	40	30	20	10	5	2.5	1.25
100	6	7	9	10	13	16	22	32	58	88	100	100
200	6	7	9	11	13	17	23	34	66	116	176	200
1000	6	7	9	11	13	17	24	36	74	145	275	501
2000	6	7	9	11	13	17	24	37	75	150	291	552
2500	6	7	9	11	13	17	24	37	75	150	297	571
5000	6	7	9	11	13	17	24	37	75	152	303	596
10000	6	7	9	11	13	17	24	37	75	152	305	607
15000	6	7	9	11	13	17	24	37	75	152	306	610
20000	6	7	9	11	13	17	24	37	75	153	307	614
25000	6	7	9	11	13	17	24	37	76	153	307	618
50000	6	7	9	11	13	17	24	37	76	155	309	619
Infinite	6	7	9	11	13	17	24	37	76	155	309	619

Table 13j: Sample Sizes for Lot Quality Assurance Sampling
No more than **4** cases acceptable with **95%** confidence

Prevalence %

Population	90	80	70	60	50	40	30	20	10	5	2.5	1.25
100	7	8	10	12	15	19	26	38	66	95	100	100
200	7	9	10	13	16	20	27	41	77	132	191	200
1000	7	9	10	13	16	20	28	43	87	170	321	578
2000	7	9	10	13	16	21	28	43	88	176	342	643
2500	7	9	10	13	16	21	28	43	89	177	349	669
5000	7	9	10	13	16	21	28	43	89	179	357	701
10000	7	9	10	13	16	21	28	44	89	180	361	715
15000	7	9	10	13	16	21	28	44	89	180	361	720
20000	7	9	10	13	16	21	28	44	89	180	362	724
25000	7	9	10	13	16	21	28	44	90	181	363	728
50000	7	9	10	13	16	21	28	44	90	181	363	728
Infinite	7	9	10	13	16	21	28	44	90	181	364	730

Table 13k: Sample Sizes for Lot Quality Assurance Sampling
No case acceptable with **90%** confidence

Prevalence %

Population	90	80	70	60	50	40	30	20	10	5	2.5	1.25
100	2	2	2	3	4	5	7	10	20	37	78	94
200	2	2	2	3	4	5	7	11	21	41	78	120
1000	2	2	2	3	4	5	7	11	22	44	87	168
2000	2	2	2	3	4	5	7	11	22	45	89	175
2500	2	2	2	3	4	5	7	11	22	45	90	177
5000	2	2	2	3	4	5	7	11	22	45	91	181
10000	2	2	2	3	4	5	7	11	22	45	91	182
15000	2	2	2	3	4	5	7	11	22	45	91	182
20000	2	2	2	3	4	5	7	11	22	45	91	184
25000	2	2	2	3	4	5	7	11	23	45	92	184
50000	2	2	2	3	4	5	7	11	23	46	92	184
Infinite	2	2	2	3	4	5	7	11	23	46	92	184

Table 13I: Sample Sizes for Lot Quality Assurance Sampling
No more than **1** case acceptable with **90%** confidence

Prevalence %

Population	90	80	70	60	50	40	30	20	10	5	2.5	1.25
100	3	4	4	5	7	8	11	17	32	56	93	100
200	3	4	4	5	7	9	12	18	35	65	112	188
1000	3	4	4	5	7	9	12	18	37	74	145	274
2000	3	4	4	5	7	9	12	18	38	76	149	290
2500	3	4	4	5	7	9	12	18	38	76	151	296
5000	3	4	4	5	7	9	12	18	38	76	153	303
10000	3	4	4	5	7	9	12	19	38	76	154	305
15000	3	4	4	5	7	9	12	19	38	76	154	308
20000	3	4	4	5	7	9	12	19	38	76	154	311
25000	3	4	4	5	7	9	12	19	38	77	155	311
50000	3	4	4	5	7	9	12	19	38	77	155	311
Infinite	3	4	4	5	7	9	12	19	38	77	155	311

Table 13m: Sample Sizes for Lot Quality Assurance Sampling
No more than **2** cases acceptable with **90%** confidence

Prevalence %

Population	90	80	70	60	50	40	30	20	10	5	2.5	1.25
100	4	5	6	7	9	12	16	23	43	71	100	100
200	4	5	6	7	9	12	16	24	47	86	141	199
1000	4	5	6	7	9	12	16	25	51	101	195	366
2000	4	5	6	7	9	12	16	25	52	104	203	391
2500	4	5	6	7	9	12	16	25	52	104	206	401
5000	4	5	6	7	9	12	16	25	52	105	209	414
10000	4	5	6	7	9	12	16	25	52	105	210	418
15000	4	5	6	7	9	12	16	25	52	105	211	420
20000	4	5	6	7	9	12	16	25	52	105	211	426
25000	4	5	6	8	9	12	17	25	52	105	212	427
50000	4	5	6	8	9	12	17	25	52	106	212	427
Infinite	4	5	6	8	9	12	17	25	52	106	212	427

Table 13n: Sample Sizes for Lot Quality Assurance Sampling
No more than **3** cases acceptable with **90%** confidence

Prevalence %

Population	90	80	70	60	50	40	30	20	10	5	2.5	1.25
100	5	6	8	9	11	14	19	29	52	82	100	100
200	5	6	8	9	12	15	20	30	58	104	164	200
1000	5	6	8	9	12	15	21	32	64	126	241	449
2000	5	6	8	9	12	15	21	32	65	130	253	484
2500	5	6	8	9	12	15	21	32	65	130	258	500
5000	5	6	8	9	12	15	21	32	65	131	262	518
10000	5	6	8	10	12	15	21	32	65	132	264	526
15000	5	6	8	10	12	15	21	32	65	132	265	527
20000	5	6	8	10	12	15	21	32	65	132	265	531
25000	5	6	8	10	12	15	21	32	66	132	267	535
50000	5	7	8	10	12	15	21	32	66	135	267	535
Infinite	5	7	8	10	12	15	21	32	66	135	267	535

Table 13o: Sample Sizes for Lot Quality Assurance Sampling
No more than **4** cases acceptable with **90%** confidence

Population	Prevalence %											
	90	80	70	60	50	40	30	20	10	5	2.5	1.25
100	7	8	9	11	14	17	23	34	60	90	100	100
200	7	8	9	11	14	18	24	36	69	121	180	200
1000	7	8	9	11	14	18	25	38	77	150	285	527
2000	7	8	9	11	14	18	25	38	78	155	302	572
2500	7	8	9	11	14	18	25	38	78	156	308	595
5000	7	8	9	11	14	18	25	38	78	157	314	619
10000	7	8	9	12	14	18	25	38	78	158	316	628
15000	7	8	10	12	14	18	25	38	78	158	316	628
20000	7	8	10	12	14	18	25	38	78	158	317	637
25000	7	8	10	12	14	18	25	38	79	159	318	637
50000	7	8	10	12	14	18	25	39	79	159	318	637
Infinite	7	8	10	12	14	18	25	39	79	159	318	638

Table 14a: Sample Size and Decision Rule for LQAS

(Level of significance: **1%**; Power: **90%**; Alternative hypothesis: **1-sided**)

$P_0\%$

$P_a\%$	50 n	50 d	55 n	55 d	60 n	60 d	65 n	65 d	70 n	70 d	75 n	75 d	80 n	80 d	85 n	85 d	90 n	90 d	95 n	95 d
5	11;	1	9;	1	7;	1	6;	1	5;	1	*		*		*		*		*	
10	15;	2	12;	2	10;	2	8;	2	6;	1	5;	1	*		*		*		*	
15	22;	5	17;	4	13;	3	10;	2	8;	2	6;	2	5;	1	*		*		*	
20	32;	9	23;	7	18;	5	13;	4	10;	3	8;	3	6;	2	5;	2	*		*	
25	48;	15	33;	11	24;	8	18;	6	13;	5	10;	4	8;	3	6;	3	*		*	
30	77;	28	49;	18	34;	13	24;	10	18;	8	13;	6	10;	5	7;	3	5;	2	*	
35	140;	56	79;	33	50;	21	33;	15	23;	10	17;	8	12;	6	9;	5	6;	3	5;	3
40	321;	139	142;	64	79;	37	49;	24	32;	16	22;	11	16;	9	11;	6	8;	5	6;	4
45	1298;	607	323;	156	141;	71	77;	40	47;	25	31;	17	21;	12	14;	8	9;	6	7;	5
50			1294;	670	317;	169	137;	76	73;	41	44;	26	28;	17	18;	11	12;	8	9;	7
55					1264;	717	306;	179	129;	78	68;	42	40;	26	24;	16	15;	10	11;	8
60							1208;	746	287;	182	119;	78	61;	41	35;	24	20;	14	14;	11
65									1126;	752	262;	180	106;	75	52;	38	28;	21	20;	16
70											1018;	731	231;	170	90;	68	42;	33	29;	24
75													883;	678	192;	151	70;	57	47;	41
80															722;	591	147;	123	94;	84
85																	535;	465		

* Sample size less than 5

Table 14b: Sample Size and Decision Rule for LQAS
(Level of significance: **1%**; Power: **80%**; Alternative hypothesis: **1-sided**)

$P_0\%$

$P_a\%$	50 n	50 d	55 n	55 d	60 n	60 d	65 n	65 d	70 n	70 d	75 n	75 d	80 n	80 d	85 n	85 d	90 n	90 d	95 n	95 d
5	9	1	8	1	6	0	5	0	*	*	*	*	*	*	*	*	*	*	*	*
10	13	2	10	1	8	1	7	1	5	1	*	*	*	*	*	*	*	*	*	*
15	18	4	14	3	11	2	8	2	7	2	5	1	*	*	*	*	*	*	*	*
20	25	6	19	5	14	4	11	3	8	2	6	2	5	1	*	*	*	*	*	*
25	38	11	26	8	19	6	14	4	11	4	8	3	6	2	*	*	*	*	*	*
30	60	20	39	14	26	9	19	7	14	5	10	4	7	3	5	2	*	*	*	*
35	109	42	61	24	38	15	26	11	18	8	13	6	9	4	7	3	*	*	*	*
40	249	106	110	48	61	27	38	17	25	12	17	8	12	6	8	4	5	2	*	*
45	1001	463	249	118	108	52	59	29	36	18	23	12	15	8	10	5	7	4	*	*
50			997	511	244	128	105	56	56	31	33	18	21	12	13	8	8	5	5	3
55					972	547	234	135	98	58	51	31	30	18	18	11	11	7	6	4
60							927	568	219	137	90	57	46	30	25	17	14	9	7	5
65									862	572	199	135	79	54	38	27	20	14	10	7
70											777	554	174	126	66	49	30	23	13	10
75													671	512	143	111	51	40	19	15
80															546	444	108	89	32	27
85																	399	345	66	58

Table 14c: Sample Size and Decision Rule for LQAS
(Level of significance: **1%**; Power: **50%**; Alternative hypothesis: **1-sided**)

P0%

Pa%	50 n	50 d	55 n	55 d	60 n	60 d	65 n	65 d	70 n	70 d	75 n	75 d	80 n	80 d	85 n	85 d	90 n	90 d	95 n	95 d
5	7	0	6	0	5	0	*		*		*		*		*		*		*	
10	9	1	7	0	6	0	5	0	*		*		*		*		*		*	
15	12	1	9	1	7	1	5	0	*		*		*		*		*		*	
20	16	3	11	2	9	1	7	1	5	1	*		*		*		*		*	
25	22	5	15	3	11	2	8	2	6	1	5	1	*		*		*		*	
30	34	10	22	6	15	4	11	3	8	2	6	2	*		*		*		*	
35	61	21	34	11	21	7	14	4	10	3	7	2	5	1	*		*		*	
40	136	54	60	24	33	13	20	8	13	5	9	3	6	2	*		*		*	
45	542	243	134	60	58	26	31	13	19	8	12	5	8	3	5	2	*		*	
50			536	268	130	65	55	27	29	14	17	8	10	5	6	3	*		*	
55					520	286	124	68	51	28	26	14	14	7	8	4	*		*	
60							493	295	114	68	46	27	22	13	12	7	6	3	*	
65									455	295	102	66	39	25	18	11	8	5	*	
70											406	284	87	60	31	21	13	9	5	3
75													347	260	69	51	22	16	7	5
80															276	220	49	39	12	9
85																	195	165	26	22

* Sample size less than 5

Table 14d: Sample Size and Decision Rule for LQAS

(Level of significance: **5%**; Power: **90%**; Alternative hypothesis: **1-sided**)

$P_0\%$

$P_a\%$	50 n ; d	55 n ; d	60 n ; d	65 n ; d	70 n ; d	75 n ; d	80 n ; d	85 n ; d	90 n ; d	95 n ; d
5	6 ; 0	5 ; 0	*	*	*	*	*	*	*	*
10	10 ; 2	8 ; 2	6 ; 1	5 ; 1	*	*	*	*	*	*
15	14 ; 3	11 ; 3	8 ; 2	7 ; 2	5 ; 1	*	*	*	*	*
20	20 ; 6	15 ; 5	11 ; 3	9 ; 3	7 ; 2	5 ; 2	*	*	*	*
25	31 ; 10	21 ; 7	16 ; 6	12 ; 5	9 ; 4	7 ; 3	5 ; 2	*	*	*
30	50 ; 19	32 ; 12	22 ; 9	16 ; 7	12 ; 5	9 ; 4	7 ; 3	5 ; 2	*	*
35	92 ; 38	52 ; 22	33 ; 15	22 ; 10	16 ; 8	11 ; 5	8 ; 4	6 ; 3	5 ; 3	*
40	211 ; 93	93 ; 43	52 ; 25	32 ; 16	22 ; 11	15 ; 8	11 ; 6	8 ; 5	6 ; 4	*
45	853 ; 402	212 ; 104	93 ; 48	51 ; 27	31 ; 17	21 ; 12	14 ; 8	10 ; 6	7 ; 4	*
50		852 ; 444	210 ; 114	91 ; 51	49 ; 29	30 ; 18	19 ; 12	13 ; 8	9 ; 6	5 ; 3
55			834 ; 477	203 ; 120	87 ; 53	46 ; 29	27 ; 18	17 ; 12	11 ; 8	7 ; 5
60				798 ; 496	191 ; 123	80 ; 53	42 ; 29	24 ; 17	14 ; 10	8 ; 6
65					746 ; 501	176 ; 122	72 ; 52	36 ; 27	20 ; 15	11 ; 9
70						676 ; 488	156 ; 116	62 ; 48	30 ; 24	15 ; 12
75							589 ; 455	131 ; 104	49 ; 40	21 ; 18
80								484 ; 398	102 ; 86	34 ; 30
85									362 ; 316	67 ; 60

* Sample size less than 5

Table 14e: Sample Size and Decision Rule for LQAS

(Level of significance: **5%**;   Power: **80%**;   Alternative hypothesis: **1-sided**)

P₀%

Pa%	50 n	50 d	55 n	55 d	60 n	60 d	65 n	65 d	70 n	70 d	75 n	75 d	80 n	80 d	85 n	85 d	90 n	90 d	95 n	95 d
5	5	0	5	0	*		*		*		*		*		*		*		*	
10	8	1	6	1	5	1	*		*		*		*		*		*		*	
15	11	2	8	2	7	2	5	1	*		*		*		*		*		*	
20	15	4	11	3	9	2	7	2	5	1	*		*		*		*		*	
25	23	7	16	5	12	4	9	3	7	2	5	2	*		*		*		*	
30	37	13	24	9	16	6	12	5	9	4	6	2	5	2	*		*		*	
35	67	26	38	15	24	10	16	7	11	5	8	3	6	3	*		*		*	
40	153	66	68	30	38	17	23	11	16	8	11	5	8	4	5	2	*		*	
45	617	288	154	74	67	33	37	19	22	11	15	8	10	5	7	4	5	3	*	
50			615	317	151	80	65	35	35	20	21	12	13	8	9	5	6	4	*	
55					600	340	145	84	62	37	32	19	19	12	12	8	7	4	*	
60							573	353	136	86	57	37	29	19	16	11	10	7	5	3
65									534	356	125	85	50	35	25	18	13	9	7	5
70											483	346	109	80	43	32	20	15	9	7
75													419	321	91	71	33	26	14	11
80															342	279	69	58	22	19
85																	253	219	44	39

* Sample size less than 5

Table 14f: Sample Size and Decision Rule for LQAS
(Level of significance: 5%; Power: 50%; Alternative hypothesis: 1-sided)

$P_0\%$

$P_a\%$	50 n	50 d	55 n	55 d	60 n	60 d	65 n	65 d	70 n	70 d	75 n	75 d	80 n	80 d	85 n	85 d	90 n	90 d	95 n	95 d
5	*		*		*		*		*		*		*		*		*		*	
10	5	0	*		*		*		*		*		*		*		*		*	
15	6	0	5	0	*		*		*		*		*		*		*		*	
20	8	1	6	1	5	1	*		*		*		*		*		*		*	
25	11	2	8	2	6	1	*		*		*		*		*		*		*	
30	17	5	11	3	8	2	6	1	*		*		*		*		*		*	
35	31	10	17	5	11	3	7	2	5	1	*		*		*		*		*	
40	68	27	30	12	17	6	10	4	7	2	5	2	*		*		*		*	
45	271	121	67	30	29	13	16	7	10	4	6	2	5	2	*		*		*	
50			268	134	65	32	28	14	15	7	9	4	7	3	*		*		*	
55					260	143	62	34	26	14	13	7	11	6	6	3	*		*	
60							247	148	57	34	23	13	20	13	9	5	*		*	
65									228	148	51	33	44	30	16	11	7	4	*	
70											203	142	174	130	35	26	11	8	*	
75															138	110	25	20	*	
80																	98	83	6	4
85																			13	11

* Sample size less than 5

Table 14g: Sample Size and Decision Rule for LQAS
(Level of significance: **10%**; Power: **90%**; Alternative hypothesis: **1-sided**)

P₀%

Pₐ%	50 n	50 d	55 n	55 d	60 n	60 d	65 n	65 d	70 n	70 d	75 n	75 d	80 n	80 d	85 n	85 d	90 n	90 d	95 n	95 d
5	5	1	*		*		*		*		*		*		*		*		*	
10	7	1	6	1	5	1	*		*		*		*		*		*		*	
15	10	2	8	2	6	2	5	1	*		*		*		*		*		*	
20	15	5	11	3	9	3	7	2	5	2	*		*		*		*		*	
25	23	8	16	6	12	5	9	4	7	3	5	2	*		*		*		*	
30	38	15	25	10	17	7	12	5	9	4	7	3	5	2	*		*		*	
35	70	29	39	17	25	11	17	8	12	6	9	5	7	4	5	3	*		*	
40	161	72	72	34	40	20	25	13	17	9	12	7	9	5	6	3	5	3	*	
45	654	310	163	81	72	37	39	21	25	14	16	9	11	7	8	5	6	4	*	
50			654	343	161	88	70	40	38	22	23	14	15	10	10	7	7	5	5	4
55					641	368	156	93	67	42	36	23	22	15	14	10	9	6	6	5
60							615	384	148	96	63	42	33	23	19	14	12	9	7	5
65									575	388	137	96	57	41	29	22	16	12	9	7
70											522	378	121	91	49	38	24	19	13	11
75													456	353	103	82	40	33	18	15
80															377	311	81	69	28	25
85																	284	249	55	50

* Sample size less than 5

Table 14h: Sample Size and Decision Rule for LQAS
(Level of significance: **10%**; Power: **80%**; Alternative hypothesis: **1-sided**)

$P_0\%$

$P_a\%$	50 (n ; d)	55 (n ; d)	60 (n ; d)	65 (n ; d)	70 (n ; d)	75 (n ; d)	80 (n ; d)	85 (n ; d)	90 (n ; d)	95 (n ; d)
5	*	*	*	*	*	*	*	*	*	*
10	5 ; 1	*	*	*	*	*	*	*	*	*
15	8 ; 2	6 ; 1	5 ; 1	*	*	*	*	*	*	*
20	11 ; 3	8 ; 2	6 ; 2	5 ; 1	*	*	*	*	*	*
25	17 ; 5	12 ; 4	9 ; 3	6 ; 2	5 ; 2	*	*	*	*	*
30	27 ; 10	17 ; 6	12 ; 5	9 ; 4	6 ; 2	5 ; 2	*	*	*	*
35	49 ; 20	27 ; 11	17 ; 7	12 ; 5	8 ; 3	6 ; 3	5 ; 2	*	*	*
40	111 ; 48	49 ; 22	28 ; 13	17 ; 8	12 ; 6	8 ; 4	6 ; 3	*	*	*
45	450 ; 211	112 ; 54	49 ; 25	27 ; 14	17 ; 9	11 ; 6	8 ; 4	5 ; 3	*	*
50		449 ; 233	110 ; 59	48 ; 26	26 ; 15	16 ; 9	10 ; 6	7 ; 4	5 ; 3	*
55			439 ; 250	107 ; 63	45 ; 27	24 ; 15	14 ; 9	9 ; 6	6 ; 4	*
60				420 ; 260	100 ; 64	42 ; 27	22 ; 15	13 ; 9	8 ; 6	*
65					392 ; 262	92 ; 63	38 ; 27	19 ; 14	10 ; 7	6 ; 5
70						354 ; 255	81 ; 60	32 ; 24	15 ; 12	8 ; 6
75							308 ; 237	68 ; 54	25 ; 20	11 ; 9
80								253 ; 207	53 ; 44	17 ; 14
85									188 ; 163	34 ; 30

* Sample size less than 5

Table 14i: Sample Size and Decision Rule for LQAS

(Level of significance: **10%**; Power: **50%**; Alternative hypothesis: **1-sided**)

P₀% → $P_0\%$

$P_a\%$	50 n	50 d	55 n	55 d	60 n	60 d	65 n	65 d	70 n	70 d	75 n	75 d	80 n	80 d	85 n	85 d	90 n	90 d	95 n	95 d
5	*		*		*		*		*		*		*		*		*		*	
10	*		*		*		*		*		*		*		*		*		*	
15	*		*		*		*		*		*		*		*		*		*	
20	5	1	*		*		*		*		*		*		*		*		*	
25	7	1	5	1	*		*		*		*		*		*		*		*	
30	11	3	7	2	5	1	5	1	*		*		*		*		*		*	
35	19	6	11	3	7	2	6	2	*		*		*		*		*		*	
40	42	16	19	7	10	4	10	4	*		*		*		*		*		*	
45	165	74	41	18	18	8	17	8	6	2	*		*		*		*		*	
50			163	81	40	20	38	20	9	4	5	2	*		*		*		*	
55					158	86	150	90	16	8	8	4	5	2	*		*		*	
60									35	21	14	8	7	4	*		*		*	
65									138	89	31	20	12	7	6	3	*		*	
70											124	86	27	18	10	7	*		*	
75													106	79	21	15	7	5	*	
80															84	67	15	12	*	
85																	60	51	8	6

* Sample size less than 5

Table 15: Sample Size to Estimate the Incidence Rate to within ε percent, with **99%**, **95%** or **90%** Confidence Level

ε	99%	95%	90%
0.01	66358	38417	27061
0.02	16590	9605	6766
0.03	7374	4269	3007
0.04	4148	2402	1692
0.05	2655	1537	1083
0.06	1844	1068	752
0.07	1355	785	553
0.08	1037	601	423
0.09	820	475	335
0.10	664	385	271
0.12	461	267	188
0.14	339	197	139
0.16	260	151	106
0.18	205	119	84
0.20	166	97	68
0.22	138	80	56
0.24	116	67	47
0.26	99	57	41
0.28	85	50	35
0.30	74	43	31
0.32	65	38	27
0.34	58	34	24
0.36	52	30	21
0.38	46	27	19
0.40	42	25	17
0.42	38	22	16
0.44	35	20	14
0.46	32	19	13
0.48	29	17	12
0.50	27	16	11

Table 16a: Sample Size for One-Sample Test of Incidence Density

(Level of significance: 1%;   Power: 90%;   Alternative hypothesis: 2-sided)

λ_0

λ_a	0.05	0.10	0.15	0.20	0.25	0.30	0.35	0.40	0.45	0.50	0.55	0.60	0.65	0.70	0.75	0.80	0.85	0.90	0.95
0.05		42	21	15	13	12	11	10	10	10	9	9	9	9	9	9	8	8	8
0.10	27		106	42	27	21	17	15	14	13	12	12	11	11	11	10	10	10	10
0.15	11	81		201	70	42	30	24	21	18	17	15	14	14	13	13	12	12	11
0.20	7	27	166		325	106	60	42	33	27	23	21	19	17	16	15	15	14	13
0.25	6	15	50	280		479	150	82	55	42	34	29	25	23	21	19	18	17	16
0.30	5	11	27	81	424		662	201	106	70	52	42	35	30	27	24	22	21	19
0.35	*	8	18	42	120	597		876	259	135	88	64	51	42	36	32	28	26	24
0.40	*	7	13	27	60	166	801		1119	325	166	106	77	60	49	42	37	33	29
0.45	*	6	11	20	38	81	219	1034		1392	398	201	127	91	70	57	48	42	37
0.50	*	6	9	15	27	50	106	280	1297		1694	479	239	150	106	82	66	55	48
0.55	*	5	8	13	21	35	65	134	348	1589		2027	567	280	174	123	94	75	63
0.60	*	5	7	11	17	27	45	81	166	424	1912		2389	662	325	201	141	106	85
0.65	*	*	6	9	14	22	34	56	100	200	507	2264		2781	765	373	229	159	120
0.70	*	*	6	8	12	18	27	42	68	120	239	597	2646		3203	876	424	259	179
0.75	*	*	6	8	11	15	22	33	50	81	142	280	695	3058		3654	993	479	291
0.80	*	*	5	8	10	13	19	27	39	60	96	166	325	801	3499		4136	1119	537
0.85	*	*	5	7	9	12	16	23	32	47	70	112	192	372	914	3971		4647	1251
0.90	*	*	5	6	8	11	14	20	27	38	54	81	128	219	424	1034	4472		5187
0.95	*	*	5	6	8	10	13	17	23	32	44	63	93	147	249	478	1162	5003	

* Sample size less than 5

Table 16b: Sample Size for One-Sample Test of Incidence Density
(Level of significance: **1%**; Power: **80%**; Alternative hypothesis: **2-sided**)

λ_0

λ_a	0.05	0.10	0.15	0.20	0.25	0.30	0.35	0.40	0.45	0.50	0.55	0.60	0.65	0.70	0.75	0.80	0.85	0.90	0.95
0.05		36	19	14	12	11	10	10	10	9	9	9	9	9	8	8	8	8	8
0.10	19		89	36	24	19	16	14	13	12	12	11	11	10	10	10	10	10	9
0.15	7	59		165	60	36	27	22	19	17	15	14	13	13	12	12	11	11	11
0.20	*	19	124		264	89	51	36	29	24	21	19	17	16	15	14	14	13	13
0.25	*	10	36	211		387	124	69	47	36	30	26	23	21	19	18	17	16	15
0.30	*	7	19	59	322		533	165	89	60	45	36	31	27	24	22	20	19	18
0.35	*	5	12	30	89	456		703	212	112	74	55	44	36	31	28	25	23	21
0.40	*	*	9	19	43	124	614		896	264	137	89	65	51	43	36	32	29	26
0.45	*	*	7	13	27	59	164	795		1112	323	165	106	77	60	49	42	36	32
0.50	*	*	6	10	19	36	78	211	999		1352	387	196	124	89	69	56	47	41
0.55	*	*	5	8	14	25	47	100	264	1227		1614	457	229	144	102	79	64	53
0.60	*	*	*	7	11	19	32	59	124	322	1478		1901	533	264	165	117	89	72
0.65	*	*	*	6	9	15	24	40	73	150	386	1753		2210	615	303	188	132	100
0.70	*	*	*	5	8	12	19	30	49	89	179	456	2050		2543	703	344	212	148
0.75	*	*	*	5	7	10	15	23	36	59	105	211	532	2372		2900	796	387	237
0.80	*	*	*	*	6	9	13	19	28	43	70	124	246	614	2716		3280	896	433
0.85	*	*	*	*	6	8	11	16	22	33	51	82	143	282	702	3084		3683	1001
0.90	*	*	*	*	5	7	10	13	19	27	39	59	95	164	322	795	3475		4109
0.95	*	*	*	*	5	6	9	12	16	22	31	45	69	109	187	364	894	3890	

* Sample size less than 5

Table 16c: Sample Size for One-Sample Test of Incidence Density

(Level of significance: **1%**;   Power: **50%**;   Alternative hypothesis: **2-sided**)

λ_a \ λ_0	0.05	0.10	0.15	0.20	0.25	0.30	0.35	0.40	0.45	0.50	0.55	0.60	0.65	0.70	0.75	0.80	0.85	0.90	0.95
0.05		27	15	12	11	10	10	9	9	9	9	8	8	8	8	8	8	8	8
0.10	7		60	27	19	15	14	12	11	11	10	10	10	10	9	9	9	9	9
0.15	*	27		107	42	27	21	17	15	14	13	12	12	11	11	11	10	10	10
0.20	*	7	60		166	60	37	27	22	19	17	15	14	14	13	12	12	11	11
0.25	*	*	15	107		239	82	48	34	27	23	20	18	17	15	15	14	13	13
0.30	*	*	7	27	166		326	107	60	42	33	27	23	21	19	17	16	15	15
0.35	*	*	*	12	42	239		425	135	74	51	39	32	27	24	21	20	18	17
0.40	*	*	*	7	19	60	326		538	166	90	60	45	37	31	27	24	22	20
0.45	*	*	*	5	11	27	82	425		664	201	107	71	53	42	35	30	27	24
0.50	*	*	*	*	7	15	37	107	538		803	239	125	82	60	48	40	34	30
0.55	*	*	*	*	5	10	21	48	135	664		956	281	145	94	68	54	44	38
0.60	*	*	*	*	*	7	14	27	60	166	803		1122	326	166	107	77	60	49
0.65	*	*	*	*	*	5	10	17	34	74	201	956		1301	374	189	120	86	67
0.70	*	*	*	*	*	*	7	12	22	42	90	239	1122		1494	425	214	135	96
0.75	*	*	*	*	*	*	5	9	15	27	51	107	281	1301		1699	480	239	150
0.80	*	*	*	*	*	*	*	7	11	19	33	60	125	326	1494		1918	538	267
0.85	*	*	*	*	*	*	*	6	9	14	23	39	71	145	374	1699		2150	599
0.90	*	*	*	*	*	*	*	5	7	11	17	27	45	82	166	425	1918		2396
0.95	*	*	*	*	*	*	*	*	6	9	13	20	32	53	94	189	480	2150	

* Sample size less than 5

Table 16d: Sample Size for One-Sample Test of Incidence Density

(Level of significance: **5%**; Power: **90%**; Alternative hypothesis: **2-sided**)

λ_0

λ_a	0.05	0.10	0.15	0.20	0.25	0.30	0.35	0.40	0.45	0.50	0.55	0.60	0.65	0.70	0.75	0.80	0.85	0.90	0.95
0.05	21	28	13	10	8	7	7	6	6	6	6	6	5	5	5	5	5	5	5
0.10	9	61	72	28	17	13	11	10	9	8	8	7	7	7	7	6	6	6	6
0.15	6	21	122	137	47	28	20	16	13	12	11	10	9	9	8	8	8	7	7
0.20	6	12	38	204	223	72	40	28	21	17	15	13	12	11	10	10	9	9	8
0.25	5	9	21	61	306	331	102	55	37	28	22	19	16	15	13	12	11	11	10
0.30	*	7	14	32	89	430	459	137	72	47	35	28	23	20	17	16	14	13	12
0.35	*	6	11	21	45	122	575	608	178	91	59	43	33	28	24	21	18	17	15
0.40	*	5	9	16	29	61	160	741	779	223	113	72	52	40	33	28	24	21	19
0.45	*	5	8	12	21	38	79	204	928	970	274	137	86	61	47	38	32	28	24
0.50	*	5	7	10	16	27	49	99	252	1136	1182	331	163	102	72	55	44	37	31
0.55	*	*	6	9	13	21	34	61	122	306	1365	1416	392	192	119	83	63	50	42
0.60	*	*	6	8	11	17	26	42	74	147	366	1615	1670	459	223	137	95	72	57
0.65	*	*	5	7	10	14	21	32	51	89	174	430	1886	1946	531	257	157	108	81
0.70	*	*	5	7	9	12	17	25	38	61	104	204	500	2179	2242	608	293	178	122
0.75	*	*	5	6	8	11	15	21	30	45	71	122	236	575	2492	2560	691	331	200
0.80	*	*	*	6	8	10	14	18	25	35	53	83	140	270	656	2826	2898	779	371
0.85	*	*	*	5	7	9	13	16	21	29	41	61	95	160	306	741	3181	3258	872
0.90	*	*	*	5	7	9	12	15	19	26	33	47	69	108	181	345	832	3557	3639
0.95	*	*	*	5	6	8	11	14	18	24	27	38	55	81	122	181	345	920	

* Sample size less than 5

Table 16e: Sample Size for One-Sample Test of Incidence Density
(Level of significance: **5%**;   Power: **80%**;   Alternative hypothesis: **2-sided**)

λ_0

λ_a	0.05	0.10	0.15	0.20	0.25	0.30	0.35	0.40	0.45	0.50	0.55	0.60	0.65	0.70	0.75	0.80	0.85	0.90	0.95
0.05		23	12	9	8	7	6	6	6	6	6	5	5	5	5	5	5	5	5
0.10	14		58	23	15	12	10	9	8	8	7	7	7	6	6	6	6	6	6
0.15	6	42		108	38	23	17	14	12	10	10	9	8	8	8	7	7	7	7
0.20	*	14	86		174	58	33	23	18	15	13	12	11	10	9	9	8	8	8
0.25	*	8	26	146		256	81	44	30	23	19	16	14	13	12	11	10	10	9
0.30	*	6	14	42	221		353	108	58	38	29	23	20	17	15	14	13	12	11
0.35	*	*	9	21	62	312		466	139	73	48	35	28	23	20	18	16	15	13
0.40	*	*	7	14	31	86	419		595	174	89	58	42	33	27	23	20	18	16
0.45	*	*	6	10	19	42	114	541		739	213	108	69	50	38	31	27	23	21
0.50	*	*	5	8	14	26	55	146	680		899	256	128	81	58	44	36	30	26
0.55	*	*	*	6	11	18	34	70	181	834		1075	302	150	94	67	51	41	34
0.60	*	*	*	6	9	14	23	42	86	221	1003		1188	353	174	108	76	58	46
0.65	*	*	*	5	7	11	17	29	52	104	265	1188		1389	407	199	123	86	65
0.70	*	*	*	*	6	9	14	21	35	62	124	312	1389		1606	466	227	139	97
0.75	*	*	*	*	6	8	11	17	26	42	74	146	364	1606		1936	528	256	156
0.80	*	*	*	*	5	7	10	14	20	31	50	86	169	419	1839		2190	595	286
0.85	*	*	*	*	5	6	8	12	16	24	36	58	99	194	478	2087		2460	665
0.90	*	*	*	*	*	6	7	10	14	19	28	42	67	114	221	541	2350		2746
0.95	*	*	*	*	*	5	7	9	12	16	23	32	48	76	129	250	609	2630	

* Sample size less than 5

Table 16f: Sample Size for One-Sample Test of Incidence Density

(Level of significance: **5%**; Power: **50%**; Alternative hypothesis: **2-sided**)

λ_0

λ_a	0.05	0.10	0.15	0.20	0.25	0.30	0.35	0.40	0.45	0.50	0.55	0.60	0.65	0.70	0.75	0.80	0.85	0.90	0.95
0.05	*	16	9	7	7	6	6	6	5	5	5	5	5	5	5	5	5	5	5
0.10	*	*	35	16	11	9	8	7	7	7	6	6	6	6	6	6	5	5	5
0.15	*	16	*	62	25	16	12	10	9	8	8	7	7	7	7	6	6	6	6
0.20	*	*	35	*	97	35	21	16	13	11	10	9	9	8	8	7	7	7	7
0.25	*	*	9	62	*	139	48	28	20	16	13	12	11	10	9	9	8	8	8
0.30	*	*	*	16	97	*	189	62	35	25	19	16	14	12	11	10	10	9	9
0.35	*	*	*	7	25	139	*	246	78	43	30	23	19	16	14	13	12	11	10
0.40	*	*	*	*	11	35	189	*	312	97	52	35	26	21	18	16	14	13	12
0.45	*	*	*	*	7	16	48	246	*	385	117	62	41	31	25	21	18	16	14
0.50	*	*	*	*	*	9	21	62	312	*	465	139	73	48	35	28	23	20	18
0.55	*	*	*	*	*	6	12	28	78	385	*	554	163	84	55	40	31	26	22
0.60	*	*	*	*	*	*	8	16	35	97	465	*	650	189	97	62	45	35	29
0.65	*	*	*	*	*	*	6	10	20	43	117	554	*	753	217	110	70	50	39
0.70	*	*	*	*	*	*	*	7	13	25	52	139	650	*	865	246	124	78	56
0.75	*	*	*	*	*	*	*	6	9	16	30	62	163	753	*	984	278	139	87
0.80	*	*	*	*	*	*	*	*	7	11	19	35	73	189	865	*	1111	312	155
0.85	*	*	*	*	*	*	*	*	5	8	13	23	41	84	217	984	*	1245	347
0.90	*	*	*	*	*	*	*	*	*	7	10	16	26	48	97	246	1111	*	1387
0.95	*	*	*	*	*	*	*	*	*	5	8	12	19	31	55	110	278	1245	*

* Sample size less than 5

Table 16g: Sample Size for One-Sample Test of Incidence Density
(Level of significance: **10%**; Power: **90%**; Alternative hypothesis: **2-sided**)

λ_0

λ_a	0.05	0.10	0.15	0.20	0.25	0.30	0.35	0.40	0.45	0.50	0.55	0.60	0.65	0.70	0.75	0.80	0.85	0.90	0.95
0.05		21	10	7	6	5	5	5	5	*	*	*	*	*	*	*	*	*	*
0.10	18		57	21	13	10	8	7	7	6	6	5	5	5	5	5	5	5	5
0.15	8	51		109	37	21	15	12	10	9	8	7	7	6	6	6	6	6	6
0.20	6	18	102		179	57	31	21	16	13	12	10	9	8	8	7	7	8	8
0.25	5	11	33	169		266	81	43	29	21	17	14	13	11	10	9	9	8	8
0.30	*	8	18	51	254		369	109	57	37	27	21	18	15	13	12	11	10	9
0.35	*	7	13	27	74	356		490	142	72	46	33	26	21	18	16	14	13	12
0.40	*	6	10	18	38	102	474		629	179	90	57	41	31	25	21	19	16	15
0.45	*	5	8	14	25	51	133	610		764	220	109	68	48	37	30	25	21	19
0.50	*	5	7	11	18	33	66	169	784		934	266	130	81	57	43	34	29	24
0.55	*	*	6	9	14	23	42	83	209	934		1146	315	154	94	66	50	39	33
0.60	*	*	6	8	12	18	29	51	102	254	1121		1352	369	179	109	76	57	45
0.65	*	*	5	7	10	15	23	36	62	122	303	1326		1576	428	206	125	86	64
0.70	*	*	5	7	9	13	18	27	43	74	145	356	1548		1817	490	235	142	97
0.75	*	*	5	6	8	11	15	22	33	51	88	169	413	1786		2075	557	266	160
0.80	*	*	5	6	7	10	13	18	26	38	60	102	196	474	2042		2351	629	298
0.85	*	*	*	5	7	9	12	16	21	30	45	70	117	224	540	2315		2643	704
0.90	*	*	*	5	6	8	10	13	18	25	35	51	80	133	254	610	2606		2952
0.95	*	*	*	5	6	7	9	12	16	21	29	40	59	90	151	286	685	2913	

* Sample size less than 5

Table 16h: Sample Size for One-Sample Test of Incidence Density
(Level of significance: **10%**; Power: **80%**; Alternative hypothesis: **2-sided**)

λ_0

λ_a	0.05	0.10	0.15	0.20	0.25	0.30	0.35	0.40	0.45	0.50	0.55	0.60	0.65	0.70	0.75	0.80	0.85	0.90	0.95
0.05	12	18	9	7	6	5	5	5	*	*	*	*	*	*	*	*	*	*	*
0.10	5	34	44	18	11	9	7	7	6	6	5	5	5	5	5	5	*	*	*
0.15	*	12	69	83	29	18	13	10	9	8	7	7	6	6	6	5	5	5	5
0.20	*	7	21	117	135	44	25	18	14	11	10	9	8	7	7	7	6	6	6
0.25	*	5	12	34	177	199	62	34	23	18	14	12	11	10	9	8	8	7	7
0.30	*	*	8	18	50	249	275	83	44	29	22	18	15	13	11	10	10	9	8
0.35	*	*	6	12	25	69	334	364	108	56	36	27	21	18	15	13	12	11	10
0.40	*	*	5	9	16	34	92	431	465	135	69	44	32	25	21	18	15	14	12
0.45	*	*	*	7	12	21	45	117	540	578	165	83	53	38	29	24	20	18	16
0.50	*	*	*	6	9	15	27	56	145	662	704	199	99	62	44	34	28	23	20
0.55	*	*	*	5	7	12	19	34	69	177	796	842	235	116	72	51	39	31	26
0.60	*	*	*	*	6	9	15	24	42	84	211	942	992	275	135	83	58	44	35
0.65	*	*	*	*	5	8	12	18	29	50	100	249	1101	1155	318	155	95	66	50
0.70	*	*	*	*	*	7	10	14	21	34	60	117	290	1272	1330	364	176	108	75
0.75	*	*	*	*	*	6	8	12	17	25	40	69	136	334	1456	1518	412	199	121
0.80	*	*	*	*	*	5	7	10	14	20	30	47	80	155	381	1652	1718	465	223
0.85	*	*	*	*	*	*	6	9	12	16	23	34	54	92	177	431	1860	1930	520
0.90	*	*	*	*	*	*	*	8	10	13	19	27	39	61	104	199	484	2081	2154
0.95	*	*	*	*	*	*	*	*	*	*	*	*	*	*	*	*	*	*	*

* Sample size less than 5

Table 16i: Sample Size for One-Sample Test of Incidence Density
(Level of significance: **10%**; Power: **50%**; Alternative hypothesis: **2-sided**)

λ_0

λ_a	0.05	0.10	0.15	0.20	0.25	0.30	0.35	0.40	0.45	0.50	0.55	0.60	0.65	0.70	0.75	0.80	0.85	0.90	0.95
0.05	*	11	7	5	5	*	*	*	*	*	*	*	*	*	*	*	*	*	*
0.10	*	*	25	11	8	7	6	5	5	5	5	*	*	*	*	*	*	*	*
0.15	*	11	*	44	17	11	9	7	7	6	6	5	5	5	5	5	*	*	*
0.20	*	*	25	*	68	25	15	11	9	8	7	7	6	6	6	5	5	5	5
0.25	*	*	7	44	*	98	34	20	14	11	10	8	8	7	7	6	6	6	5
0.30	*	*	*	11	68	*	133	44	25	17	14	11	10	9	8	7	7	7	6
0.35	*	*	*	5	17	98	*	174	55	31	21	16	13	11	10	9	8	8	7
0.40	*	*	*	*	8	25	133	*	220	68	37	25	19	15	13	11	10	9	9
0.45	*	*	*	*	5	11	34	174	*	271	82	44	29	22	17	15	13	11	10
0.50	*	*	*	*	*	7	15	44	220	*	328	98	51	34	25	20	16	14	13
0.55	*	*	*	*	*	*	9	20	55	271	*	390	115	59	39	28	22	18	16
0.60	*	*	*	*	*	*	6	11	25	68	328	*	458	133	68	44	32	25	20
0.65	*	*	*	*	*	*	*	7	14	31	82	390	*	531	153	77	49	36	28
0.70	*	*	*	*	*	*	*	5	9	17	37	98	458	*	609	174	87	55	40
0.75	*	*	*	*	*	*	*	*	7	11	21	44	115	531	*	693	196	98	62
0.80	*	*	*	*	*	*	*	*	5	8	14	25	51	133	609	*	783	220	109
0.85	*	*	*	*	*	*	*	*	*	6	10	16	29	59	153	693	*	877	245
0.90	*	*	*	*	*	*	*	*	*	5	7	11	19	34	68	174	783	*	977
0.95	*	*	*	*	*	*	*	*	*	*	6	8	13	22	39	77	196	877	*

* Sample size less than 5

Table 17a: Sample Size for Test of Equality of Incidence Densities

(Level of significance: **1%**; Power: **90%**; Alternative hypothesis: **2-sided**)

λ_0

λ_a	0.05	0.10	0.15	0.20	0.25	0.30	0.35	0.40	0.45	0.50	0.55	0.60	0.65	0.70	0.75	0.80	0.85	0.90	0.95
0.05		70	33	24	20	17	16	15	14	14	13	13	13	13	12	12	12	12	12
0.10	70		189	70	43	33	27	24	21	20	18	17	17	16	16	15	15	14	14
0.15	33	189		368	122	70	49	39	33	29	26	24	22	21	20	19	18	17	17
0.20	24	70	368		606	189	103	70	53	43	37	33	29	27	25	24	22	21	20
0.25	20	43	122	606		903	271	143	94	70	56	47	41	36	33	30	28	26	25
0.30	17	33	70	189	903		1261	368	189	122	89	70	58	49	43	39	35	33	30
0.35	16	27	49	103	271	1261		1677	479	242	154	110	86	70	59	52	46	41	38
0.40	15	24	39	70	143	368	1677		2154	606	301	189	134	103	83	70	60	53	48
0.45	14	21	33	53	94	189	479	2154		2690	747	368	228	160	122	98	82	70	61
0.50	14	20	29	43	70	122	242	606	2690		3285	903	440	271	189	143	114	94	80
0.55	13	18	26	37	56	89	154	301	747	3285		3940	1075	520	317	220	165	131	108
0.60	13	17	24	33	47	70	110	189	368	903	3940		4654	1261	606	368	253	189	149
0.65	13	17	22	29	41	58	86	134	228	440	1075	4654		5428	1462	698	422	289	215
0.70	13	16	21	27	36	49	70	103	160	271	520	1261	5428		6262	1677	798	479	327
0.75	12	16	20	25	33	43	59	83	122	189	317	606	1462	6262		7155	1908	903	541
0.80	12	15	19	24	30	39	52	70	98	143	220	368	698	1677	7155		8107	2154	1016
0.85	12	15	18	22	28	35	46	60	82	114	165	253	422	798	1908	8107		9120	2414
0.90	12	14	17	21	26	33	41	53	70	94	131	189	289	479	903	2154	9120		10191
0.95	12	14	17	20	25	30	38	48	61	80	108	149	215	327	541	1016	2414	10191	

Table 17b: Sample Size for Test of Equality of Incidence Densities
(Level of significance: **1%**; Power: **80%**; Alternative hypothesis: **2-sided**)

λ_0

λ_a	0.05	0.10	0.15	0.20	0.25	0.30	0.35	0.40	0.45	0.50	0.55	0.60	0.65	0.70	0.75	0.80	0.85	0.90	0.95
0.05		54	25	18	15	13	12	11	11	11	10	10	10	10	9	9	9	9	9
0.10	54		148	54	34	25	21	18	16	15	14	13	13	12	12	11	11	11	11
0.15	25	148		288	95	54	38	30	25	22	20	18	17	16	15	14	14	13	13
0.20	18	54	288		475	148	80	54	41	34	29	25	23	21	19	18	17	16	16
0.25	15	34	95	475		709	212	112	73	54	43	36	31	28	25	23	22	20	19
0.30	13	25	54	148	709		989	288	148	95	69	54	45	38	34	30	27	25	23
0.35	12	21	38	80	212	989		1316	376	190	120	86	67	54	46	40	36	32	29
0.40	11	18	30	54	112	288	1316		1690	475	236	148	105	80	65	54	47	41	37
0.45	11	16	25	41	73	148	376	1690		2111	586	288	179	126	95	76	64	54	48
0.50	11	15	22	34	54	95	190	475	2111		2578	709	345	212	148	112	89	73	63
0.55	10	14	20	29	43	69	120	236	586	2578		3092	843	408	249	172	129	102	84
0.60	10	13	18	25	36	54	86	148	288	709	3092		3653	989	475	288	198	148	116
0.65	10	13	17	23	31	45	67	105	179	345	843	3653		4260	1147	548	331	226	168
0.70	10	13	16	21	28	38	54	80	126	212	408	989	4260		4915	1316	626	376	256
0.75	9	12	15	19	25	34	46	65	95	148	249	475	1147	4915		5615	1497	709	424
0.80	9	11	14	18	23	30	40	54	76	112	172	288	548	1316	5615		6363	1690	797
0.85	9	11	14	17	22	27	36	47	64	89	129	198	331	626	1497	6363		7158	1895
0.90	9	11	13	16	20	25	32	41	54	73	102	148	226	376	709	1690	7158		7999
0.95	9	11	13	16	19	23	29	37	48	63	84	116	168	256	424	797	1895	7999	

Table 17c: Sample Size for Test of Equality of Incidence Densities
(Level of significance: **1%**; Power: **50%**; Alternative hypothesis: **2-sided**)

λ_0

λ_a	0.05	0.10	0.15	0.20	0.25	0.30	0.35	0.40	0.45	0.50	0.55	0.60	0.65	0.70	0.75	0.80	0.85	0.90	0.95
0.05		30	14	10	8	7	6	6	6	5	5	5	5	5	5	5	5	5	5
0.10	30		83	30	19	14	11	10	9	8	7	7	7	6	6	6	6	6	6
0.15	14	83		163	54	30	21	17	14	12	11	10	9	8	8	8	7	7	7
0.20	10	30	163		269	83	45	30	23	19	16	14	12	11	10	10	9	9	8
0.25	8	19	54	269		402	120	63	41	30	24	20	17	15	14	13	12	11	10
0.30	7	14	30	83	402		561	163	83	54	39	30	25	21	19	17	15	14	13
0.35	6	11	21	45	120	561		747	213	107	68	48	37	30	26	22	20	18	16
0.40	6	10	17	30	63	163	747		959	269	134	83	59	45	36	30	26	23	20
0.45	6	9	14	23	41	83	213	959		1198	332	163	101	71	54	43	36	30	27
0.50	5	8	12	19	30	54	107	269	1198		1464	402	196	120	83	63	50	41	35
0.55	5	7	11	16	24	39	68	134	332	1464		1756	478	231	141	97	73	57	47
0.60	5	7	10	14	20	30	48	83	163	402	1756		2074	561	269	163	112	83	66
0.65	5	7	9	12	17	25	37	59	101	196	478	2074		2419	651	311	187	128	95
0.70	5	6	8	11	15	21	30	45	71	120	231	561	2419		2791	747	355	213	145
0.75	5	6	8	10	14	19	26	36	54	83	141	269	651	2791		3189	850	402	240
0.80	5	6	8	10	13	17	22	30	43	63	97	163	311	747	3189		3614	959	452
0.85	5	6	7	9	12	15	20	26	36	50	73	112	187	355	850	3614		4065	1075
0.90	5	6	7	9	11	14	18	23	30	41	57	83	128	213	402	959	4065		4543
0.95	5	6	7	8	10	13	16	20	27	35	47	66	95	145	240	452	1075	4543	

Table 17d: Sample Size for Test of Equality of Incidence Densities
(Level of significance: 5%;   Power: **90%**;   Alternative hypothesis: **2-sided**)

λ_0

λ_a	0.05	0.10	0.15	0.20	0.25	0.30	0.35	0.40	0.45	0.50	0.55	0.60	0.65	0.70	0.75	0.80	0.85	0.90	0.95
0.05		50	24	17	14	13	12	11	11	10	10	10	10	9	9	9	9	9	9
0.10	50		134	50	31	24	20	17	15	14	13	13	12	12	11	11	11	11	10
0.15	24	134		260	87	50	35	28	24	21	19	17	16	15	14	14	13	13	12
0.20	17	50	260		428	134	73	50	38	31	27	24	21	20	18	17	16	15	15
0.25	14	31	87	428		638	192	101	67	50	40	34	29	26	24	22	20	19	18
0.30	13	24	50	134	638		891	260	134	87	63	50	41	35	31	28	25	24	22
0.35	12	20	35	73	192	891		1185	339	171	109	78	61	50	42	37	33	30	27
0.40	11	17	28	50	101	260	1185		1521	428	213	134	95	73	59	50	43	38	34
0.45	11	15	24	38	67	134	339	1521		1900	528	260	162	114	87	70	58	50	44
0.50	10	14	21	31	50	87	171	428	1900		2320	638	311	192	134	101	81	67	57
0.55	10	13	19	27	40	63	109	213	528	2320		2783	759	368	225	156	117	93	76
0.60	10	13	17	24	34	50	78	134	260	638	2783		3287	891	428	260	179	134	106
0.65	10	12	16	21	29	41	61	95	162	311	759	3287		3834	1033	494	298	205	152
0.70	9	12	15	20	26	35	50	73	114	192	368	891	3834		4422	1185	564	339	231
0.75	9	11	14	18	24	31	42	59	87	134	225	428	1033	4422		5053	1348	638	382
0.80	9	11	14	17	22	28	37	50	70	101	156	260	494	1185	5053		5726	1521	718
0.85	9	11	13	16	20	25	33	43	58	81	117	179	298	564	1348	5726		6440	1705
0.90	9	11	13	15	19	24	30	38	50	67	93	134	205	339	638	1521	6440		7197
0.95	9	10	12	15	18	22	27	34	44	57	76	106	152	231	382	718	1705	7197	

Table 17e: Sample Size for Test of Equality of Incidence Densities
(Level of significance: **5%**; Power: **80%**; Alternative hypothesis: **2-sided**)

λ_0

λ_a	0.05	0.10	0.15	0.20	0.25	0.30	0.35	0.40	0.45	0.50	0.55	0.60	0.65	0.70	0.75	0.80	0.85	0.90	0.95
0.05		37	17	13	10	9	9	8	8	7	7	7	7	7	7	7	7	6	6
0.10	37		100	37	23	17	14	13	11	10	10	9	9	9	8	8	8	8	8
0.15	17	100		194	64	37	26	21	17	15	14	13	12	11	10	10	10	9	9
0.20	13	37	194		320	100	54	37	28	23	20	17	16	14	13	13	12	11	11
0.25	10	23	64	320		477	143	75	50	37	30	25	22	19	17	16	15	14	13
0.30	9	17	37	100	477		665	194	100	64	47	37	31	26	23	21	19	17	16
0.35	9	14	26	54	143	665		885	253	128	81	58	45	37	31	27	24	22	20
0.40	8	13	21	37	75	194	885		1136	320	159	100	71	54	44	37	32	28	25
0.45	8	11	17	28	50	100	253	1136		1419	394	194	120	85	64	52	43	37	32
0.50	7	10	15	23	37	64	128	320	1419		1733	477	232	143	100	75	60	50	42
0.55	7	10	14	20	30	47	81	159	394	1733		2078	567	274	168	116	87	69	57
0.60	7	9	13	17	25	37	58	100	194	477	2078		2455	665	320	194	134	100	79
0.65	7	9	12	16	22	31	45	71	120	232	567	2455		2863	771	369	222	153	113
0.70	7	9	11	14	19	26	37	54	85	143	274	665	2863		3303	885	421	253	173
0.75	7	8	10	13	17	23	31	44	64	100	168	320	771	3303		3774	1007	477	285
0.80	7	8	10	13	16	21	27	37	52	75	116	194	369	885	3774		4277	1136	536
0.85	7	8	10	12	15	19	24	32	43	60	87	134	222	421	1007	4277		4811	1274
0.90	6	8	9	11	14	17	22	28	37	50	69	100	153	253	477	1136	4811		5376
0.95	6	8	9	11	13	16	20	25	32	42	57	79	113	173	285	536	1274	5376	

Table 17f: Sample Size for Test of Equality of Incidence Densities
(Level of significance: **5%**; Power: **50%**; Alternative hypothesis: **2-sided**)

λ_0

λ_a	0.05	0.10	0.15	0.20	0.25	0.30	0.35	0.40	0.45	0.50	0.55	0.60	0.65	0.70	0.75	0.80	0.85	0.90	0.95
0.05		18	8	6	5	*	*	*	*	*	*	*	*	*	*	*	*	*	*
0.10	18		49	18	11	8	7	6	6	5	5	*	*	*	*	*	*	*	*
0.15	8	49		95	31	18	13	10	8	7	6	6	5	5	5	5	*	*	5
0.20	6	18	95		156	49	26	18	13	11	9	8	7	7	6	6	6	5	5
0.25	5	11	31	156		233	70	37	24	18	14	12	10	9	8	8	7	7	6
0.30	*	8	18	49	233		325	95	49	31	23	18	15	13	11	10	10	8	8
0.35	*	7	13	26	70	325		433	123	62	39	28	22	18	15	13	12	10	10
0.40	*	6	10	18	37	95	433		556	156	78	49	34	26	21	18	15	13	12
0.45	*	6	8	13	24	49	123	556		694	193	95	59	41	31	25	21	18	16
0.50	*	5	7	11	18	31	62	156	694		848	233	113	70	49	37	29	24	20
0.55	*	5	6	9	14	23	39	78	193	848		1017	277	134	82	57	42	33	28
0.60	*	*	6	8	12	18	28	49	95	233	1017		1201	325	156	95	65	49	38
0.65	*	*	5	7	10	15	22	34	59	113	277	1201		1401	377	180	109	74	55
0.70	*	*	5	7	9	13	18	26	41	70	134	325	1401		1616	433	206	123	84
0.75	*	*	5	6	8	11	15	21	31	49	82	156	377	1616		1846	492	233	139
0.80	*	*	5	6	8	10	13	18	25	37	57	95	180	433	1846		2092	556	262
0.85	*	*	*	6	7	10	12	15	21	29	42	65	109	206	492	2092		2353	623
0.90	*	*	*	5	7	8	10	13	18	24	33	49	74	123	233	556	2353		2630
0.95	*	*	5	5	6	8	10	12	16	20	28	38	55	84	139	262	623	2630	

* Sample size less than 5

Table 17g: Sample Size for Test of Equality of Incidence Densities
(Level of significance: 10%; Power: 90%; Alternative hypothesis: 2-sided)

λ_a \ λ_0	0.05	0.10	0.15	0.20	0.25	0.30	0.35	0.40	0.45	0.50	0.55	0.60	0.65	0.70	0.75	0.80	0.85	0.90	0.95
0.05		41	19	14	12	11	10	9	9	9	8	8	8	8	8	8	8	8	8
0.10	41		109	41	26	19	16	14	13	12	11	11	10	10	10	9	9	9	9
0.15	19	109		212	71	41	29	23	19	17	15	14	13	13	12	11	11	11	10
0.20	14	41	212		349	109	60	41	31	26	22	19	18	16	15	14	13	13	12
0.25	12	26	71	349		521	157	83	55	41	33	28	24	21	19	18	17	16	15
0.30	11	19	41	109	521		726	212	109	71	52	41	34	29	26	23	21	19	18
0.35	10	16	29	60	157	726		966	277	140	89	64	50	41	35	30	27	24	22
0.40	9	14	23	41	83	212	966		1240	349	174	109	78	60	49	41	35	31	28
0.45	9	13	19	31	55	109	277	1240		1549	431	212	132	93	71	57	48	41	36
0.50	9	12	17	26	41	71	140	349	1549		1891	521	254	157	109	83	66	55	47
0.55	8	11	15	22	33	52	89	174	431	1891		2268	619	300	183	127	96	76	63
0.60	8	11	14	19	28	41	64	109	212	521	2268		2680	726	349	212	146	109	86
0.65	8	10	13	18	24	34	50	78	132	254	619	2680		3125	842	403	243	167	124
0.70	8	10	13	16	21	29	41	60	93	157	300	726	3125		3605	966	460	277	189
0.75	8	10	12	15	19	26	35	49	71	109	183	349	842	3605		4119	1099	521	312
0.80	8	9	11	14	18	23	30	41	57	83	127	212	403	966	4119		4667	1240	585
0.85	8	9	11	13	17	21	27	35	48	66	96	146	243	460	1099	4667		5250	1390
0.90	8	9	11	13	16	19	24	31	41	55	76	109	167	277	521	1240	5250		5867
0.95	8	9	10	12	15	18	22	28	36	47	63	86	124	189	312	585	1390	5867	

Table 17h: Sample Size for Test of Equality of Incidence Densities
(Level of significance: **10%**; Power: **80%**; Alternative hypothesis: **2-sided**)

λ_0

λ_a	0.05	0.10	0.15	0.20	0.25	0.30	0.35	0.40	0.45	0.50	0.55	0.60	0.65	0.70	0.75	0.80	0.85	0.90	0.95
0.05		29	14	10	8	8	7	7	6	6	6	6	6	6	5	5	5	5	5
0.10	29		79	29	18	14	12	10	9	8	8	8	7	7	7	7	6	6	6
0.15	14	79		153	51	29	21	16	14	12	11	10	9	9	8	8	8	8	7
0.20	10	29	153		252	79	43	29	22	18	16	14	13	12	11	10	10	9	9
0.25	8	18	51	252		376	113	60	39	29	24	20	17	15	14	13	12	11	11
0.30	8	14	29	79	376		524	153	79	51	37	29	24	21	18	16	15	14	13
0.35	7	12	21	43	113	524		697	199	101	64	46	36	29	25	22	19	17	16
0.40	7	10	16	29	60	153	697		895	252	126	79	56	43	35	29	25	22	20
0.45	6	9	14	22	39	79	199	895		1118	311	153	95	67	51	41	34	29	26
0.50	6	8	12	18	29	51	101	252	1118		1365	376	183	113	79	60	48	39	34
0.55	6	8	11	16	24	37	64	126	311	1365		1638	447	216	132	92	69	55	45
0.60	6	8	10	14	20	29	46	79	153	376	1638		1934	524	252	153	106	79	62
0.65	6	7	9	13	17	24	36	56	95	183	447	1934		2256	608	291	176	120	90
0.70	6	7	9	12	15	21	29	43	67	113	216	524	2256		2602	697	332	199	136
0.75	5	7	8	11	14	18	25	35	51	79	132	252	608	2602		2974	793	376	225
0.80	5	7	8	10	13	16	22	29	41	60	92	153	291	697	2974		3369	895	422
0.85	5	6	8	10	12	15	19	25	34	48	69	106	176	332	793	3369		3790	1004
0.90	5	6	8	9	11	14	17	22	29	39	55	79	120	199	376	895	3790		4235
0.95	5	6	7	9	11	13	16	20	26	34	45	62	90	136	225	422	1004	4235	

Table 17i: Sample Size for Test of Equality of Incidence Densities
(Level of significance: **10%**; Power: **50%**; Alternative hypothesis: **2-sided**)

λ_a	\multicolumn{19}{c}{λ_0}
	0.05	0.10	0.15	0.20	0.25	0.30	0.35	0.40	0.45	0.50	0.55	0.60	0.65	0.70	0.75	0.80	0.85	0.90	0.95
0.05	*	13	6	*	*	*	*	*	*	*	*	*	*	*	*	*	*	*	*
0.10	13	*	34	13	8	6	5	*	*	*	*	*	*	*	*	*	*	*	*
0.15	6	34	*	67	22	13	9	7	6	5	5	*	*	*	*	*	*	*	*
0.20	*	13	67	*	110	34	19	13	10	8	7	6	5	5	*	*	*	*	*
0.25	*	8	22	110	*	164	49	26	17	13	10	8	7	6	5	5	5	5	5
0.30	*	6	13	34	164	*	229	67	34	22	16	13	10	9	8	7	6	6	6
0.35	*	5	9	19	49	229	*	305	87	44	28	20	16	13	11	9	8	7	7
0.40	*	*	7	13	26	67	305	*	392	110	55	34	24	19	15	13	11	10	9
0.45	*	*	6	10	17	34	87	392	*	489	136	67	41	29	22	18	15	13	11
0.50	*	*	5	8	13	22	44	110	489	*	597	164	80	49	34	26	21	17	15
0.55	*	*	5	7	10	16	28	55	136	597	*	716	195	94	58	40	30	24	20
0.60	*	*	*	6	8	13	20	34	67	164	716	*	846	229	110	67	46	34	27
0.65	*	*	*	5	7	10	16	24	41	80	195	846	*	987	266	127	77	53	39
0.70	*	*	*	5	6	9	13	19	29	49	94	229	987	*	1138	305	145	87	59
0.75	*	*	*	*	5	8	11	15	22	34	58	110	266	1138	*	1301	347	164	98
0.80	*	*	*	*	5	7	9	13	18	26	40	67	127	305	1301	*	1474	392	185
0.85	*	*	*	*	5	6	8	11	15	21	30	46	77	145	347	1474	*	1658	439
0.90	*	*	*	*	5	6	7	10	13	17	24	34	53	87	164	392	1658	*	1853
0.95	*	*	*	*	5	6	7	9	11	15	20	27	39	59	98	185	439	1853	*

* Sample size less than 5

Index